# FIRST FRCR ANATOMY
# EXAMINATION REVISION

# FIRST FRCR ANATOMY
# EXAMINATION REVISION

### Alexander J King
MBBS MRCS
*Specialty Registrar in Clinical Radiology*
*Southampton University Hospital Trust*
*Wessex Radiology Training Scheme*

and

### Benjamin J Hudson
MBBS
*Specialty Registrar in Clinical Radiology*
*Norfolk & Norwich University Hospital*
*East of England Radiology Training Scheme*

Foreword by

### Joanna Fairhurst
*Consultant Paediatric Radiologist*
*Southampton University Hospital Trust*

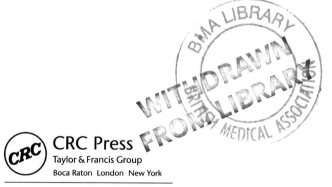

**CRC Press**
Taylor & Francis Group
Boca Raton London New York

CRC Press is an imprint of the
Taylor & Francis Group, an **informa** business

**Radcliffe Publishing Ltd**
33–41 Dallington Street
London
EC1V 0BB
United Kingdom

**www.radcliffepublishing.com**

Electronic catalogue and worldwide online ordering facility.

British Library Cataloguing in Publication Data

A catalogue record for this book is available from the British Library.

ISBN-13: 978 184619 476 4

The paper used for the text pages of this book is FSC® certified. FSC® (The Forest Stewardship Council) is an international network to promote responsible management of the world's forests.

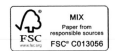

Typeset by Phoenix Photosetting, Chatham, Kent

# Contents

# Foreword

No one can deny the rapid pace at which the examination structure for the Fellowship of the Royal College of Radiologists has been changing in recent years. We barely had time to get used to the re-introduction of a standalone Physics Examination before the Multiple Choice Question format for the Part IIA modules was replaced by Single Best Answer papers. Now candidates are also faced with an Anatomy examination which, although not novel in idea, presents new challenges for a generation of radiologists in training who have already had to adapt to major changes in the Curriculum.

How should candidates prepare themselves for sitting this examination? A trite answer would be to read about and learn all the anatomy that can be identified on contemporary imaging. This is, however, an almost impossible task, and probably a counsel of perfection. One approach might be to identify those topics and areas where a sound knowledge of anatomy will be of ongoing use throughout a career in radiology: in this way the candidate is not just preparing for an examination but also laying a firm foundation for their future professional activities. Alternatively, radiologists in training may seek a more focused aid to exam preparation: this textbook satisfies both aims.

The authors have understood that radiological anatomy is not the same as surgical anatomy, and have applied this rule in identifying the necessary scope of this text, which is therefore comprehensive but not exhausting. They have sought out key images that lend themselves to five questions being set, and have ensured that the contents are sufficiently detailed and probing. The Reader can be assured that a thorough knowledge of the text will go a long way to ensuring exam success.

This textbook is the first of its kind, and will doubtless prove popular amongst radiologists in training. However, to confine its readership to these candidates would be to deny this book its greatest merit: that of serving as a handbook and revision aide for all imagers regardless of the stage of their career. Most radiologists have an affinity for attractive images and puzzle-solving, and this book allows us to indulge both passions whilst reminding us of the roots of our profession.

**Joanna Fairhurst**
**Consultant Paediatric Radiologist**
**Southampton University Hospital Trust**
*March 2011*

# Preface

The anatomy component of the FRCR examination was reintroduced in the spring of 2010. The intention was to formally assess the anatomical knowledge required to perform and interpret a variety of radiological studies. According to the Royal College of Radiology, the level of knowledge should reflect about six months of specialty training in radiology, with 30 hours of focused teaching in radiological anatomy.

The syllabus incorporates imaging in a variety of modalities, including computed tomography, magnetic resonance imaging, ultrasound, fluoroscopy and plain radiography. It also includes imaging of normal anatomical variants as well as imaging in the first trimester of pregnancy. However, the current syllabus explicitly excludes nuclear medicine studies and endoluminal ultrasound images from the examination.

Obviously we are unable to cover every single point of anatomical knowledge. There are some very fine radiological anatomy atlases available for this. Rather, in this revision aid, we have attempted to produce a collection of images that could appear in the examination. We have tried to draw from our own experience of taking the exam, as well as that of many of our colleagues, in formulating the questions for this book. These images will hopefully cover the breadth of the exam syllabus such that when faced with an image in the actual examination, you are likely to have seen the regional anatomy, imaging plane and modality before.

The examination itself consists of 20 images relating to a stem of five individual questions, totalling 100 marks overall. There are no negative marks. For the most part each image will be labelled with five arrows (A to E), and the candidate will be asked to name the structures labelled. The images are displayed on a computer screen and the candidate is able to adjust the zoom and windowing of the image. The candidate is asked to handwrite the answers in a paper booklet. On occasion they will be asked about a labelled structure or a point of anatomy relating to it (e.g. 'What is the name of the third branch of the external carotid artery?'). It is also important to note that for every question, where possible you should state the laterality of the structure (e.g. *right* adrenal gland, tendon of *left* tibialis anterior).

We have divided the book into chapters by anatomical region. This will hopefully allow you to focus your revision on a particular region (e.g. upper limb) for a period of time, and then test yourself on a series of relevant images and questions from that chapter. In addition, we have included in these chapters a number of learning points relating to the image in the question, to enhance your knowledge of radiological anatomy.

At the end of the book we have provided three mock examinations, each composed of 20 question stems and images. Under exam conditions you should allow yourself 75 minutes for each mock examination.

Finally, we wish you the best of luck with the real exam!

**Alexander J King**
**Benjamin J Hudson**
*March 2011*

# About the authors

**Alex King** qualified from Guys, King's and St Thomas's in 2004. Subsequently, he was a surgical trainee in the Wessex Deanery, where he attained MRCS in 2009. Later that year he was appointed to the Wessex Radiology Training Scheme.

**Ben Hudson** graduated from the Royal Free and University College Medical School, University College London in 2004. He went on to complete basic orthopaedic and surgical training at a number of hospitals in the London and Wessex Deaneries, before being successfully appointed to the Wessex Radiology Training Scheme in 2009. He transferred to the Norwich Training Scheme in 2010.

Alex and Ben sat and passed the First FRCR Anatomy Examination in 2010, shortly after its introduction. During that period of learning they developed and accumulated ideas that helped them to become familiar with and understand the Royal College of Radiology First FRCR Anatomy Examination curriculum. Their objective in the writing of this book has been to share some of those ideas in order to help future candidates to really understand the anatomy as it relates to radiology, rather than simply learning the images.

# List of contributors

We would like to thank all of the radiology staff at Southampton University Hospital Trust and Norfolk & Norwich University Hospital. We are particularly grateful to the following people who have contributed ideas, expertise and images:

**Dr Timothy Bryant** BMedSci BMBS MRCP FRCR
Consultant Interventional Radiologist, Southampton University Hospital Trust

**Dr Helen Oliver** BM
Specialty Registrar in Clinical Radiology, Norfolk & Norwich University Hospital

**Dr Nicholas Railton** MBBS FRCR
Consultant Interventional Radiologist, Broomfield Hospital

**Dr Ruth Walker** BSc(Hons) MBBS FRCR
Consultant Radiologist, Southampton University Hospital Trust

The illustrations were kindly provided by Daniel James, BA (Hons), Illustration student at Southampton Solent University.

To Julia and Lily for their endless patience and the immeasurable joy that they bring to my every day.

Also to Ronnie, Gillian and Vanessa for the sacrifices they made and the support they gave.

They have afforded and enabled me this opportunity.

**AK**

To
My beautiful wife Helen,
My parents Patricia and Michael for their unwavering support,
And to those who taught, inspired and encouraged me along the way: FSH, AHN and DME.

**BH**

# Chapter 1
# Head and neck

## Image 1.1

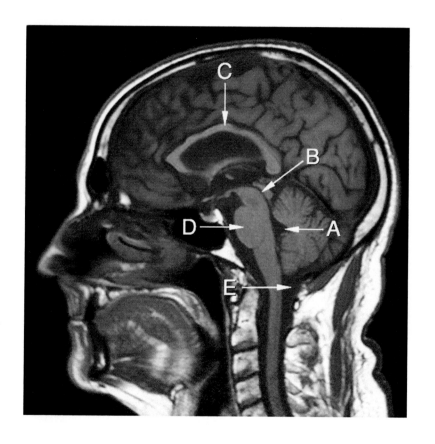

# Image: MR brain midline sagittal (1.1)

## ANSWERS

A  Fourth ventricle
B  Aqueduct of Sylvius
C  Body of corpus callosum
D  Pons
E  Cisterna magna

## LEARNING POINT

The corpus callosum provides a neural connection between the cerebral hemispheres. It is the largest white matter structure in the brain. The anterior curve is termed the genu and the posterior curve is termed the splenium, while the body connects the two. The complex third ventricle is intimately related to the corpus callosum.

The foramina of Munro are paired structures that provide a connection between the lateral ventricles and the third ventricle. The aqueduct of Sylvius provides a communication between the third and fourth ventricles. The foramen of Magendie allows cerebrospinal fluid to flow into the cisterna magna and on into the thecal sac.

**CSF flow superior to inferior**

Lateral ventricles (1 and 2)
↓
Foramina of Munro
↓
Third ventricle (3)
↓
Aqueduct of Sylvius
↓
Fourth ventricle (4)
↓
Foramen of Magendie
↓
Cisterna magna
↓
Thecal sac

Remember that it is all to do with numbers. From superior to inferior the names of the ventricles increase in magnitude: lateral (1st and 2nd ventricles), 3rd, 4th and magna (greatest).

Similarly, the number of letters in the name of the communicating ducts increases: Munro (5 letters), Sylvius (7 letters) and Magendie (8 letters).

# Image 1.2

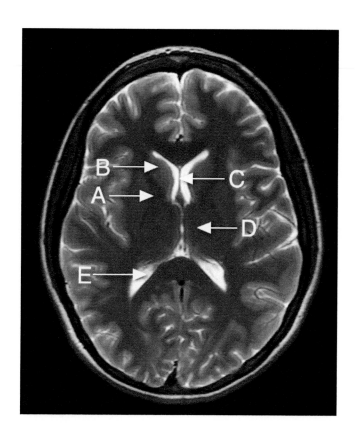

# Image: MRI brain axial (1.2)

## ANSWERS

A   Genu of right internal capsule
B   Head of right caudate nucleus
C   Septum pellucidum
D   Left thalamus
E   Trigone/posterior horn of right lateral ventricle

## LEARNING POINT

The internal capsule consists of white matter tracts that provide a connection between the cerebral cortex and the medulla. In the axial plane it separates the caudate from the lentiform nucleus and the lentiform from the thalamus.

The lateral ventricles are paired structures containing cerebrospinal fluid. The septum pellucidum is a thin membrane that separates the lateral ventricles.

# Image 1.3

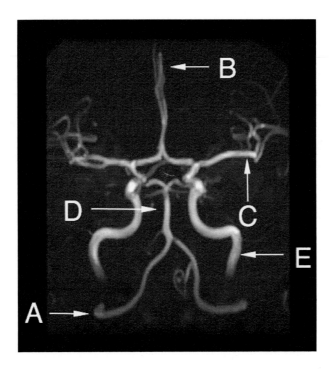

# Image: MRA circle of Willis (1.3)

## ANSWERS

A  Right vertebral artery
B  Anterior cerebral artery
C  Left middle cerebral artery
D  Basilar artery
E  Left internal carotid artery

## LEARNING POINT

The circle of Willis describes an anastomotic ring of arteries supplying blood to the brain. The vertebral arteries anastomose to form the basilar artery. The basilar artery gives off paired cerebellar vessels before dividing into the posterior cerebral arteries. The anterior and middle cerebral arteries take their origin from the internal carotid artery. The circle of Willis is completed by the anterior and posterior communicating arteries. However, this classical description is seen in less than 40% of the population.

During fetal development the posterior cerebral artery switches its main supply from the posterior communicating artery to the basilar artery as it becomes more dominant. In approximately 20% of the population the posterior cerebral artery keeps its main supply from the posterior communicating artery. The outcome of this is that in effect the internal carotid supplies the posterior cerebral artery as well as the anterior and middle branches.

# Image 1.4

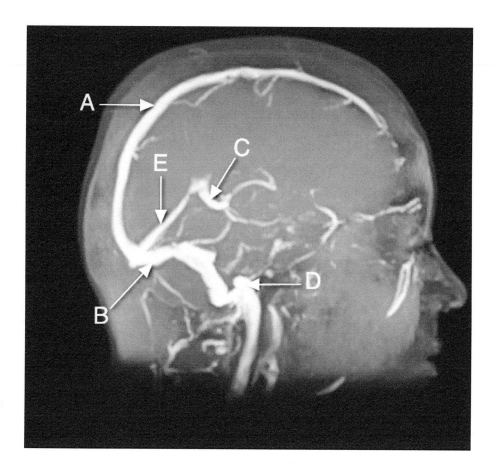

# Image: MR venogram brain (1.4)

## ANSWERS

A   Sagittal sinus
B   Transverse sinus
C   Vein of Galen
D   Jugular bulb
E   Straight sinus

## LEARNING POINT

The cerebral sinuses receive blood from the cerebral veins and cerebrospinal fluid from the subarachnoid space. They eventually all drain into the internal jugular vein. Unlike other veins they do not have valves and are encased in layers of endothelium-lined dura mater.

Unfortunately, there is no easy way to remember the names of all the veins. Labbe, Trolard, Galen and Rosenthal just have to be learned. The other veins are named anatomically, so the 'straight' is straight, and the 'sigmoid' is shaped like the Greek letter sigma.

# Image 1.5

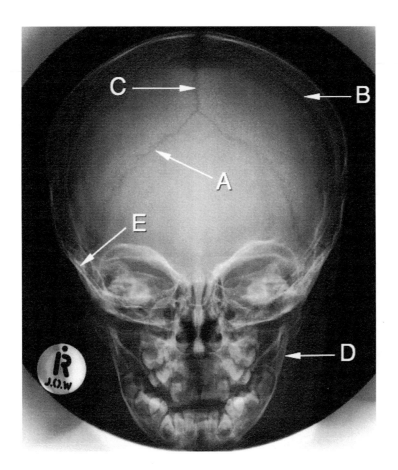

# Image: Towne's view paediatric skull (1.5)

## ANSWERS

A   Lambdoid suture
B   Coronal suture
C   Sagittal suture
D   Left side of mandible
E   Right temporal bone

## LEARNING POINT

The Towne's view typically describes an anterior–posterior radiograph taken at approximately 30 degrees.

The lambdoid sutures are easily distinguished from the coronal sutures on this view by remembering that they are named lambdoid after the Greek letter lambda, $\lambda$. The sagittal suture forms the central pole of the letter and the lambdoid sutures form the lateral limbs.

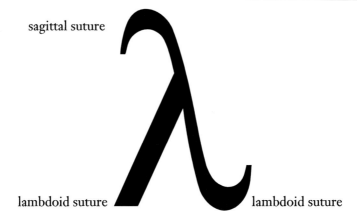

sagittal suture

lambdoid suture          lambdoid suture

# Image 1.6

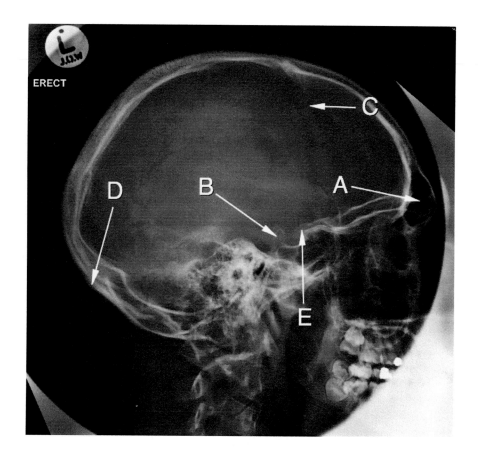

ERECT

# Image: XR skull lateral (1.6)

## ANSWERS

A    Frontal sinus
B    Dorsum sellae
C    Coronal suture
D    External occipital protuberance
E    Anterior clinoid process

## LEARNING POINT

This image helps to clarify the positions of the sutures: the lambdoid suture is posterior and the coronal suture is anterior. This image is becoming less common, but is still used as part of a skeletal survey when looking for evidence of multiple myeloma. The appearances of multiple myeloma within the skull are classically described as a 'pepperpot skull'. This refers to multiple well-defined punched-out lucencies.

The external occipital protuberance gives the attachment for the trapezius muscle, and can usually be easily palpated.

# Image 1.7

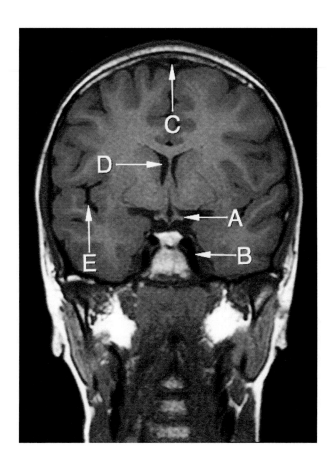

# Image: MR brain coronal (1.7)

## ANSWERS

A Left optic tract/optic chiasm
B Left internal carotid artery
C Superior sagittal sinus
D Right lateral ventricle
E Right Sylvian fissure

## LEARNING POINT

The visual pathway commences as the optic nerve and is formed behind the retina. The optic nerves pass posteriorly from the orbit through the optic foramen. The left and right optic nerves coalesce to form the optic chiasm. The fibres originating from the nasal halves of the retina cross over at the optic chiasm; the temporal portions remain on the original side of the brain. These optic tracts pass to the thalami where they terminate within the lateral geniculate nucleus. A group of axons called the optic radiation connect the lateral geniculate nuclei with the visual cortex in the posterior occipital lobe.

Remember that the optic chiasm is positioned with the pituitary gland inferior to it within the sella turcica, and the internal carotid arteries are placed laterally. Thus visual disturbance may be caused by pituitary enlargement or carotid artery aneurysm.

# Image 1.8

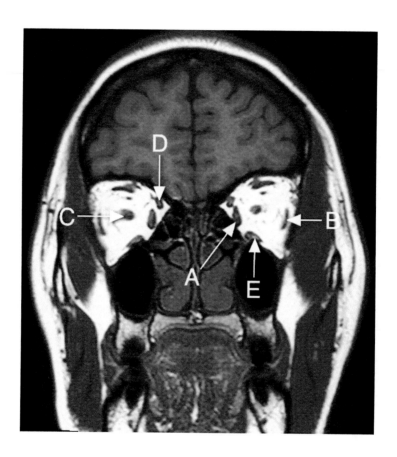

# Image: MR orbit coronal (1.8)

## ANSWERS

A  Left medial rectus
B  Left lateral rectus
C  Right optic nerve
D  Right superior oblique
E  Left inferior rectus

## LEARNING POINT

Recognition of the ocular muscles should be straightforward. They are named according to their anatomical position relative to the optic nerve, namely superior, inferior, medial, lateral and superior oblique. The lacrimal gland is positioned laterally (remember that L for lacrimal = L for lateral).

# Image 1.9

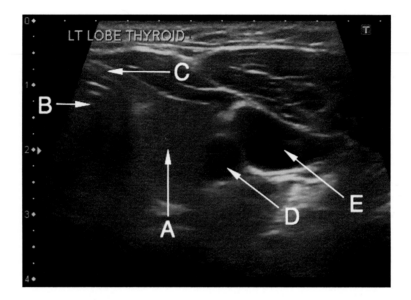

LT LOBE THYROID

# Image: US thyroid transverse (1.9)

## ANSWERS

A    Left thyroid lobe
B    Trachea
C    Thyroid isthmus
D    Left common carotid artery
E    Left jugular vein

## LEARNING POINT

The thyroid gland can be likened to a bow tie. It consists of two lateral lobes and the isthmus, which connects the lateral lobes together. An additional pyramidal lobe is sometimes seen arising anteriorly from the isthmus. The isthmus classically lies anterior to the second and third tracheal rings. The thyroid is enclosed by the pretracheal fascia and has the infrahyoid muscles overlying it anteriorly. The sternocleidomastoid muscles are positioned laterally.

The arterial supply is from the superior thyroid artery (first branch of external carotid) and the inferior thyroid artery (thyrocervical trunk from subclavian artery). There is occasionally a thyroid ima artery that arises from either the brachiocephalic artery or the aortic arch.

Venous drainage is via the superior thyroid and middle thyroid veins into the internal jugular vein, and via the inferior thyroid veins into the brachiocephalic vein.

# Image 1.10

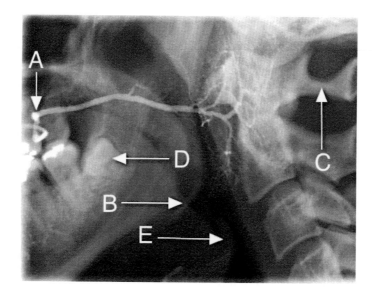

# Image: Parotid sialogram (1.10)

## ANSWERS

A   Parotid duct (Stensen's duct)
B   Angle of mandible
C   Posterior arch of atlas (C1)
D   Unerupted molar tooth
E   Epiglottis

## LEARNING POINT

The parotid gland overlies the ramus of the mandible and extends superiorly and posteriorly towards the ear. The parotid duct (Stensen's duct) opens into the oral cavity adjacent to the upper second molar tooth.

The facial nerve enters the parotid gland posteriorly and divides to give off five branches, namely the temporal, zygomatic, buccal, mandibular and cervical nerves. The external carotid artery divides into two terminal branches within the parotid gland. The branches are the superficial temporal artery and maxillary artery.

# Image 1.11

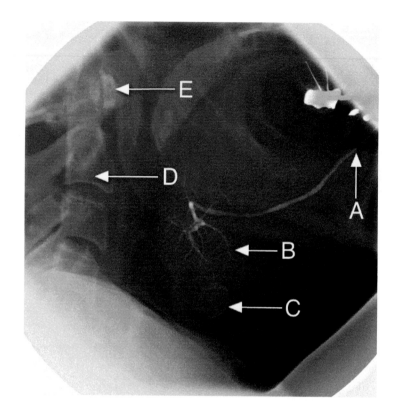

# Image: Submandibular sialogram (1.11)

## ANSWERS

A   Submandibular duct (Wharton's duct)
B   Submandibular gland
C   Hyoid bone
D   Vertebral body of axis (C2)
E   Anterior arch of atlas (C1)

## LEARNING POINT

The submandibular gland lies inferior to the mid portion of the mandible and abuts the parotid gland posteriorly. It is divided into deep and superficial portions. The submandibular gland drains into the oral cavity via Wharton's duct, which opens directly next to the frenulum on the floor of the mouth.

Notice how the submandibular gland sits inferior to the mandible, whereas the parotid gland sits posteriorly.

# Image 1.12

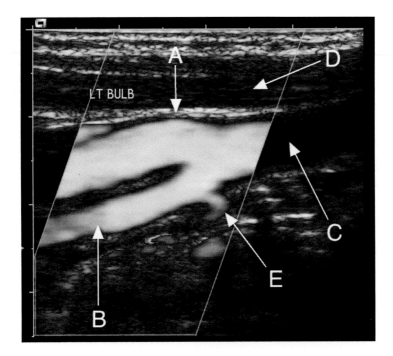

*Please refer to the colour version in the plate section.*

# Image: US Doppler carotid (1.12)

## ANSWERS

A   Internal carotid artery
B   External carotid artery
C   Common carotid artery
D   Sternocleidomastoid
E   Superior thyroid artery

## LEARNING POINT

The common carotid artery divides at the level of the fourth cervical vertebra into the internal and external carotid arteries. The internal carotid does not have any branches, and continues superiorly towards the carotid canal in the petrous temporal bone where it enters the skull.

The order of the branches of the external carotid artery can be remembered using the following mnemonic:

| | |
|---|---|
| Some | Superior thyroid |
| Anatomists | Ascending pharyngeal |
| Like | Lingual |
| Freaking | Facial |
| Out | Occipital |
| Poor | Posterior auricular |
| Medical | Maxillary |
| Students | Superficial temporal |

# Image 1.13

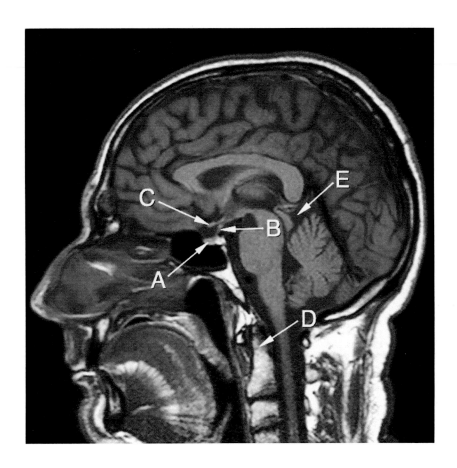

# Image: MR pituitary (1.13)

## ANSWERS

A   (Anterior) Pituitary gland
B   Infundibulum
C   Optic chiasm
D   Odontoid peg
E   Quadrigeminal cistern

## LEARNING POINT

The pituitary gland sits encased within the pituitary fossa, or sella turcica. As is seen in this sagittal image, the optic chiasm lies superior to the pituitary gland. It is clear that any enlargement of the pituitary gland is most likely to have a mass effect on the optic chiasm, as this is the only direction in which the gland is not confined. This will often give rise to a bitemporal hemianopia. The loss of the temporal fields by compression from a pituitary fossa lesion can be explained by understanding the anatomy of the visual pathway. The temporal visual field is imaged by the medial half of the retina. The medial optic tracts decussate at the optic chiasm and thus lie medially within the optic chiasm, and are therefore more likely to be compressed.

# Image 1.14

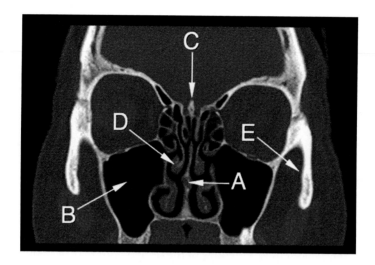

# Image: CT coronal paranasal sinuses and turbinates (1.14)

## ANSWERS

A  Nasal septum
B  Right maxillary sinus
C  Crista galli
D  Right middle turbinate
E  Left zygoma

## LEARNING POINT

The paranasal sinuses are air-filled cavities within the facial and skull bones. They are named after the bone in which they are found, and all communicate with the nasal cavity. The largest paranasal sinuses are the maxillary sinuses, and this can be appreciated on plain film radiographs. Fractures of the orbital floor may be manifested as fluid within the maxillary sinus, or orbital fat herniating through and causing a 'tear drop' to appear.

# Image 1.15

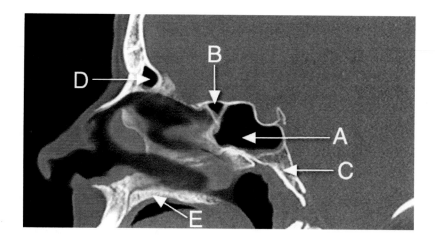

# Image: CT sagittal sphenoid sinus (1.15)

## ANSWERS

A Sphenoid sinus
B Posterior ethmoid air cells
C Clivus
D Frontal sinus
E Hard palate

## LEARNING POINT

The ethmoid air cells are a group of air-filled bony cavities that combine to form the ethmoidal sinus. Posterior to these air cells is the sphenoid sinus, which is found in the central aspect of the sphenoid bone.

The nasal turbinates divide into superior, middle and inferior components. These paired epithelium-covered bones range in size from the large inferior turbinates to the small superior turbinates.

# Image 1.16

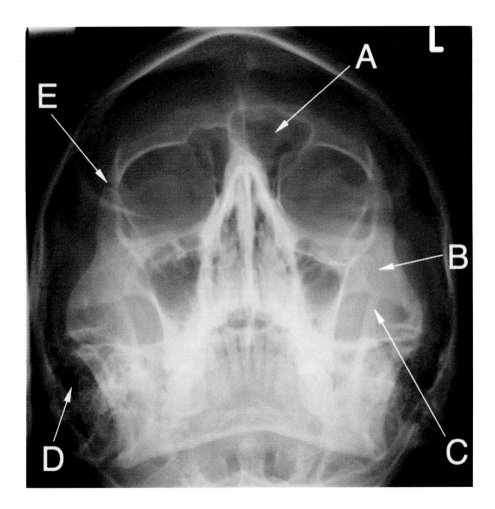

# Image: XR facial bones occipitofrontal (1.16)

## ANSWERS

A   Left frontal sinus
B   Left body of zygoma
C   Left coronoid process of mandible
D   Right mastoid process/mastoid air cells
E   Right frontozygomatic suture

## LEARNING POINT

The zygomatic bone is a complex structure with several important processes. A common fracture of the zygoma is a 'tripod' fracture. This name helps to visualise the shape of the zygoma in normal anatomy. The first, superior leg is formed by the frontal process, which continues into the frontozygomatic suture. The second, lateral leg is the temporal process of the zygoma. This process extends laterally and posteriorly to meet the zygomatic process of the temporal bone, and together they form the zygomatic arch. The inferior and lateral margins of the orbit are formed by the zygoma. Inferomedially the body of the zygoma articulates with the zygomatic process of the maxilla and maxillary sinus.

A tripod fracture will involve the floor of the orbit/maxillary sinus, the lateral margin of the orbit (with or without including the frontozygomatic suture), and the zygomatic arch.

# Image 1.17

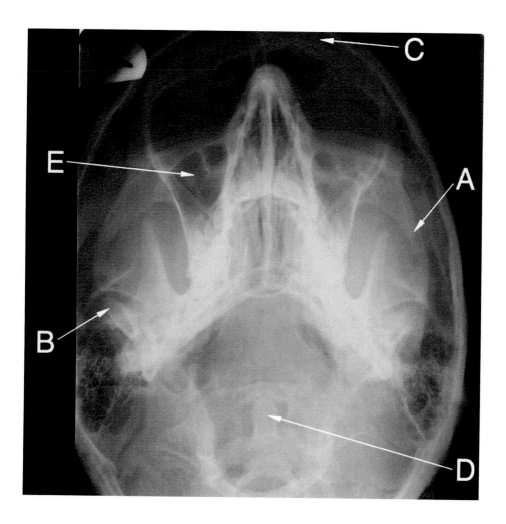

# Image: XR facial bones occipitomental (1.17)

## ANSWERS

A   Left zygomatic arch
B   Right condyle of mandible
C   Left frontal bone
D   Odontoid process/dens
E   Right maxillary sinus

## LEARNING POINT

The frontal bone contributes to several structures in the face. Primarily, the frontal bone makes up the bony structure of the entire forehead. There are two prominences just superior to the orbits called the superciliary arches. The glabella is located between these as a depression in the frontal bone. The frontal bone also contributes to the superior and supero-lateral (as the zygomatic process of the frontal bone) margins of the orbit.

# Image 1.18

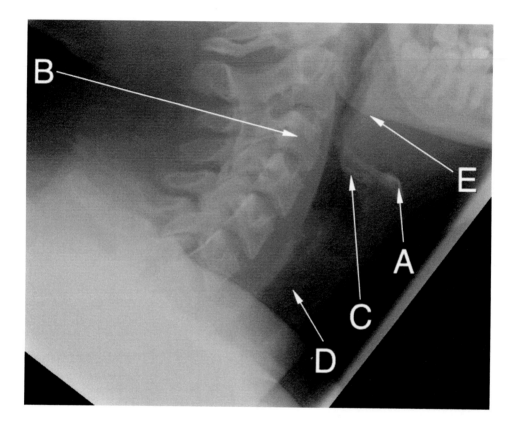

# Image: XR neck lateral (1.18)

## ANSWERS

A  Body of the hyoid bone
B  Body of the third cervical vertebra
C  Greater horn of the hyoid bone
D  Trachea/air in trachea
E  Angle of mandible

## LEARNING POINT

The hyoid bone is a 'V'-shaped bone located superiorly to the thyroid cartilage and inferiorly to the oral cavity. It consists of a central body and two laterally and posteriorly directed greater horns.

  It has no direct articulation with any other bones in the head or neck, but does form an important area of attachment for many of the muscles within the neck.

# Image 1.19

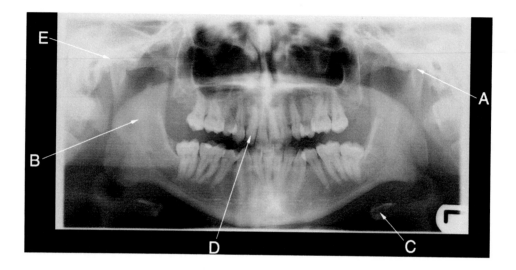

# Image: XR orthopantomogram (1.19)

## ANSWERS

A   Left condyle of mandible
B   Right ramus of mandible
C   Hyoid
D   Upper right lateral incisor
E   Right temporomandibular joint

## LEARNING POINT

The head of the mandibular condyle and the articular fossa of the temporal bone form the temporomandibular joint. The joint itself is synovial, but it is unusually divided by an articular disc splitting the joint into two halves, with two different functions. The inferior part is involved in elevation and depression of the mandible, while the superior part allows protrusion and retraction of the mandible.

The adult mouth contains different types of teeth for different purposes. The 32 adult teeth are divided into four symmetrical quadrants, each containing eight teeth (upper and lower, right and left). The most medial teeth are the incisors, which consist of the central and lateral incisors (8). Then lateral to the lateral incisors are the canines (4). Next are the first and second premolars (8), followed by the first and second molar teeth (8). Finally, most laterally and posteriorly are the wisdom teeth or third molars (4).

# Image 1.20

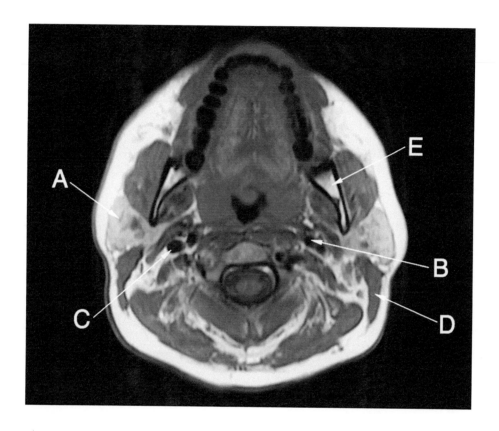

# Image: MR pharynx axial (1.20)

## ANSWERS

A   Right parotid gland
B   Left internal carotid artery
C   Right internal jugular vein
D   Left sternocleidomastoid
E   Left ramus of mandible

## LEARNING POINT

The sternocleidomastoid muscle has two origins, one arising from the manubrium of the sternum, and the other arising from the medial third of the clavicle. The two muscles merge as they ascend the anterior aspect of the neck, where the muscle inserts into the mastoid process and an aponeurotic attachment to the lateral occipital bone.

The anterior edge of the muscle forms the posterior border of the anterior triangle of the neck, which is an important surgical landmark. Its function is to tilt the head to the same side of action when working individually, and pull the head forward when working together.

# Image 1.21

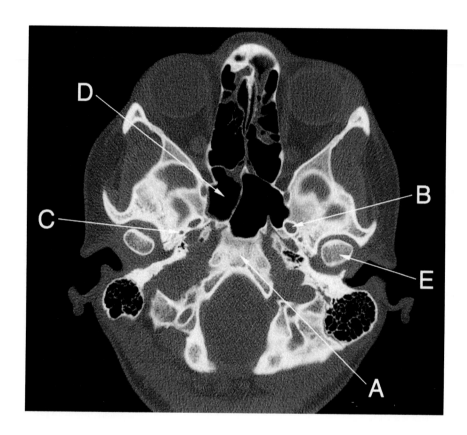

# Image: CT base of skull axial (1.21)

## ANSWERS

A   Clivus
B   Left foramen ovale
C   Right foramen spinosum
D   Sphenoid sinus
E   Left condyle of mandible

## LEARNING POINT

There are several foramina in the base of the skull that need to be recognised, as they serve as the point of exit (or entry) for several important neurological and vascular structures:

| | |
|---|---|
| **Optic canal** | Optic nerve (II) and ophthalmic artery |
| **Superior orbital fissure** | Oculomotor (III), trochlear (IV) and abducens (VI) nerves, and ophthalmic division of trigeminal nerve (Va) |
| **Foramen rotundum** | Maxillary division of trigeminal nerve (Vb) |
| **Foramen ovale** | Mandibular division of trigeminal nerve (Vc) |
| **Foramen spinosum** | Middle meningeal artery |
| **Foramen lacerum** | Internal carotid artery |
| **Foramen magnum** | Medulla oblongata/spinal cord, vertebral arteries and spinal accessory nerve (XI) |
| **Hypoglossal canal** | Hypoglossal nerve (XII) |
| **Jugular foramen** | Internal jugular vein, and glossopharyngeal (IX), vagus (X) and accessory nerves (XI) |

# Image 1.22

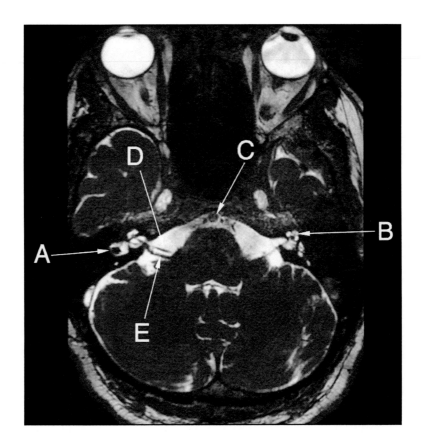

# Image: MR internal auditory meatus (1.22)

## ANSWERS

A   Right lateral semicircular canal
B   Left cochlea
C   Basilar artery
D   Right facial nerve
E   Right vestibulocochlear nerve

## LEARNING POINT

The anatomy of the inner ear is very complex! However, in simple terms the inner ear consists of three semicircular canals (lateral, posterior and superior). These connect to the vestibule, which is the central part of the labyrinth. Anterior to the vestibule is the cone-shaped cochlea.

Within the internal auditory meatus, which lies medial to the cochlea, are two of the cranial nerves. Anteriorly is the facial nerve (VII) and posteriorly is the vestibulo-cochlear nerve (VIII).

# Image 1.23

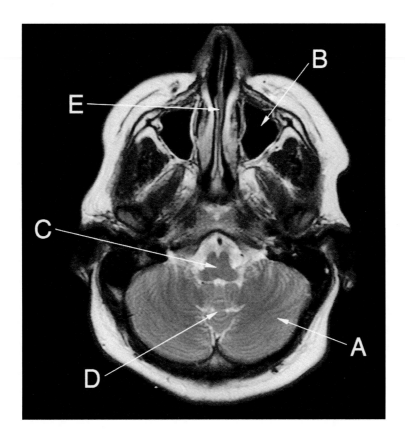

# Image: MR brain axial (1.23)

## ANSWERS

A   Left cerebellar hemisphere
B   Left maxillary sinus
C   Medulla oblongata
D   Cerebellar vermis
E   Nasal septum

## LEARNING POINT

The cerebellum is divided into left and right cerebellar hemispheres, which are joined in the midline by the cerebellar vermis (from the Latin word *vermis* meaning worm). Each hemisphere is divided into the anterior lobe, the posterior lobe and the flocculonodular lobe. The cerebellum is connected to the brainstem by three pairs of fibres known as peduncles:

*   SUPERIOR cerebellar peduncle – connecting to the **midbrain**

*   MIDDLE cerebellar peduncle – connecting to the **pons**

*   INFERIOR cerebellar peduncle – connecting to the **medulla**.

# Image 1.24

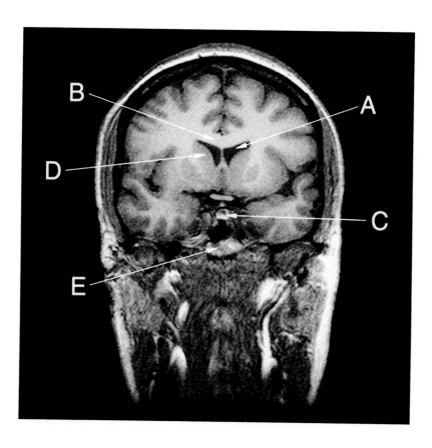

# Image: MR brain coronal (1.24)

## ANSWERS

A   Left body of lateral ventricle
B   Corpus callosum
C   Pituitary gland
D   Right head of caudate nucleus
E   Clivus

## LEARNING POINT

The clivus is formed by contributions from the basiocciput and the body of the sphenoid. It has a ramp shape (the Latin word *clivus* literally means 'slope'), which extends upwards from the anterior aspect of the foramen magnum until it reaches the dorsum sellae, which is the bony posterior boundary of the sella turcica or pituitary fossa. On either side of the clivus are the two foramina laceri, which allow the passage of the internal carotid arteries into the cranial cavity.

# Image 1.25

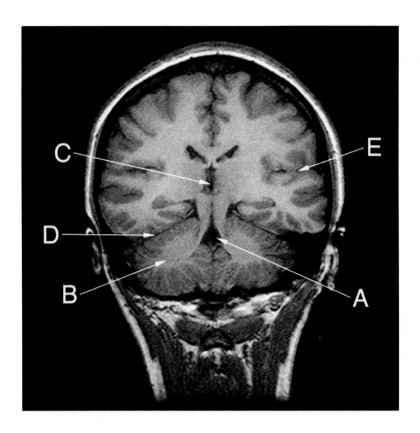

# Image: MR brain coronal (1.25)

## ANSWERS

A  Fourth ventricle
B  Right cerebellar hemisphere
C  Third ventricle
D  Right tentorium cerebelli
E  Left Sylvian fissure

## LEARNING POINT

The fourth ventricle is a diamond-shaped part of the ventricular system of the brain. The cerebellum forms the dorsal aspect of the fourth ventricle, and the lateral walls are formed by the cerebellar peduncles. The posterior aspects of the pons and medulla form the ventral margin of the ventricle. CSF enters the fourth ventricle through the aqueduct of Sylvius rostrally, and exits through the foramina of Luschka laterally, and the foramen of Magendie in the midline into the cisterna magna.

# Image 1.26

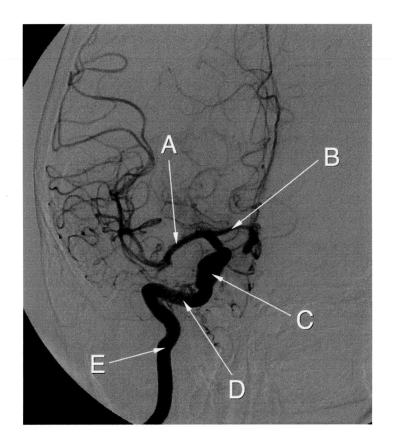

# Image: DSA internal carotid AP (1.26)

## ANSWERS

A   Middle cerebral artery
B   Anterior cerebral artery
C   Cavernous portion of internal carotid artery
D   Petrous portion of internal carotid artery
E   Cervical portion of internal carotid artery

## LEARNING POINT

The internal carotid artery arises from the common carotid artery, and ascends to the cranium inferiorly through the carotid canal and superiorly through the foramen lacerum. The artery has several named portions which follow a characteristic course, starting proximally, namely the cervical, petrous, cavernous and supraclinoid portions. The final branches of the internal carotid go to the anterior cerebral and middle cerebral arteries, as well as a contribution to the posterior communicating arteries.

# Chapter 2
# Cardiothoracic

# Image 2.1

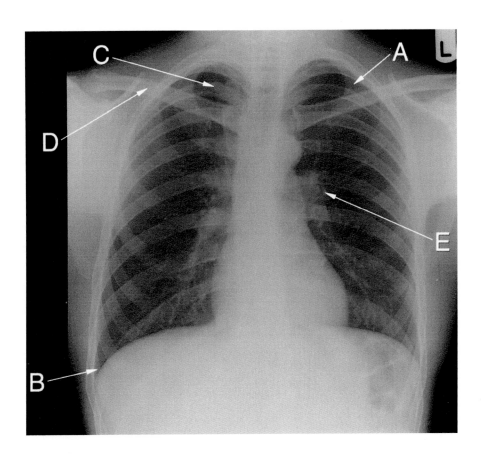

# Image: XR chest PA (2.1)

## ANSWERS

A   Left first rib
B   Right costophrenic angle
C   Azygos fissure or right posterior fourth rib
D   Right clavicle
E   Left pulmonary artery/hilum

## LEARNING POINT

An azygos fissure is an incidental finding of little consequence, formed by a laterally displaced azygos vein. The vein is enveloped by two layers of visceral and parietal pleura on each side (so there are four layers of pleura in total), giving the appearance of a relatively dense azygos fissure on a PA radiograph. The right lung medial to the fissure is termed an azygos lobe. Approximately 1% of the population have an azygos lobe.

# Image 2.2

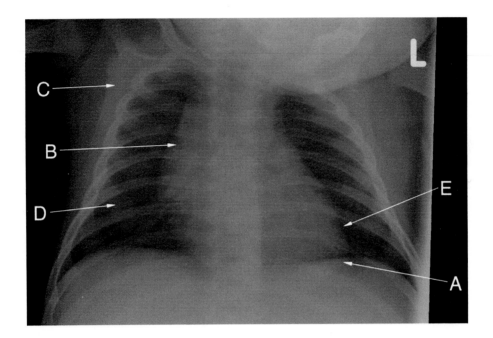

# Image: XR chest PA paediatric (2.2)

## ANSWERS

A   Left hemidiaphragm
B   Thymus
C   Right scapula
D   Right anterior fifth rib
E   Left heart border/left ventricle

## LEARNING POINT

The thymus is an organ that is usually located primarily in the superior mediastinum. It increases in size from birth to adolescence, but its relative size and weight decrease with age, and therefore the thymus appears most prominent on a radiograph during infancy. It usually consists of two lobes that meet in the midline, with the right lobe often more prominent than the left.

# Image 2.3

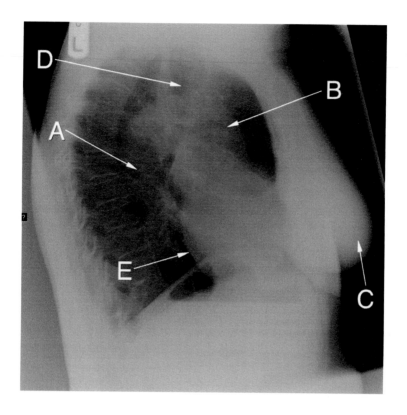

# Image: XR chest lateral (2.3)

## ANSWERS

A   Descending thoracic aorta
B   Ascending aorta
C   Breast
D   Trachea
E   Left atrial border of heart

## LEARNING POINT

The lateral chest radiograph enables visualisation of the four compartments of the mediastinum. The margins of the superior mediastinum are the thoracic inlet above, and a line drawn from the manubrio-sternal joint to the fourth thoracic vertebral body below.

Inferior to this compartment are the anterior, middle and posterior mediastinal compartments. The anterior compartment is bound by the sternum anteriorly and the pericardium and great vessels posteriorly. The majority of mediastinal masses will be located in the anterior mediastinum.

The middle mediastinum is bound by the superior, anterior and posterior mediastinal compartments, and contains the heart, the pericardium, the superior vena cava, aortic arch and ascending aorta, the main, left and right pulmonary arteries, and the distal trachea and main bronchi.

The posterior mediastinum extends from the middle mediastinum back to the anterior margin of the posterior ribs. This compartment contains the descending thoracic aorta, the azygos and hemiazygos systems, the sympathetic chains and the oesophagus.

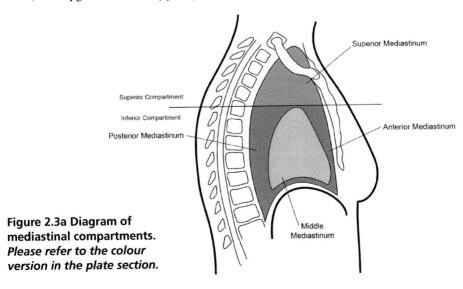

**Figure 2.3a Diagram of mediastinal compartments.** *Please refer to the colour version in the plate section.*

# Image 2.4

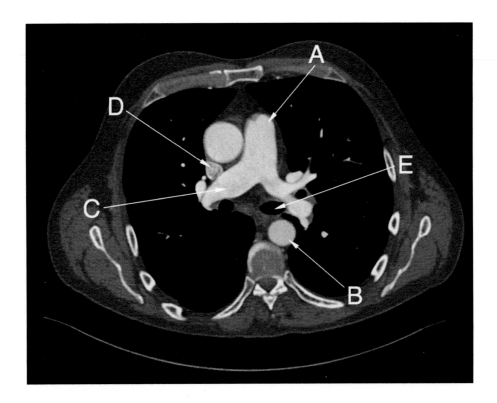

# Image: CT mediastinum axial (2.4)

## ANSWERS

A   Pulmonary trunk/main pulmonary artery
B   Descending thoracic aorta
C   Right pulmonary artery
D   Superior vena cava
E   Left main bronchus

## LEARNING POINT

The bifurcation of the main pulmonary artery occurs just to the left of the midline at the T4/5 level. The left pulmonary artery usually lies at a slightly higher level than the right. The left superior pulmonary vein passes anterior to it, with the descending aorta lying behind it.

    The right pulmonary artery is longer and more horizontal, as it has to traverse from left of the midline to reach the right lung hilum. It passes posteriorly to the ascending aorta, superior vena cava and right superior pulmonary vein. It lies in front of and slightly below the right main bronchus.

# Image 2.5

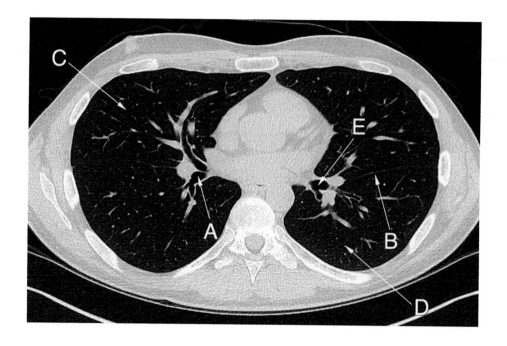

# Image: CT chest axial (2.5)

## ANSWERS

A   Right lower lobe bronchus
B   Left oblique fissure
C   Right middle lobe
D   Left lower lobe
E   Left lower lobe bronchus

## LEARNING POINT

In the right hemithorax, the horizontal fissure separates the upper lobe from the middle lobe. Anteriorly it lies at the fourth intercostal space, fanning backwards and slightly superiorly until it meets the right oblique fissure at the level of the right hilum.

The oblique fissure separates the lower lobe from the upper lobe superiorly, and the middle lobe inferiorly. Posteriorly the oblique fissure begins at about the level of the fifth thoracic vertebral body. It slopes inferiorly and anteriorly to meet its respective hemidiaphragm at the level of the sixth anterior rib.

# Image 2.6

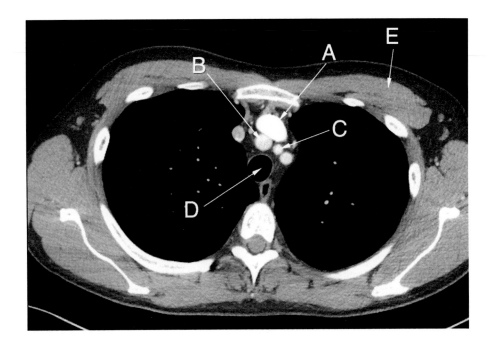

# Image: CT mediastinum axial (2.6)

## ANSWERS

A   Left brachiocephalic vein
B   Brachiocephalic trunk
C   Left common carotid artery
D   Trachea
E   Left pectoralis major

## LEARNING POINT

Three major arterial branches arise from the aortic arch, and they supply the head and neck and the upper limbs. The first branch is the brachiocephalic trunk, which soon divides into the right subclavian and right common carotid arteries. The brachiocephalic trunk is the most anterior of the three branches.

   The next branch is the left common carotid artery, which arises from the arch posterior and to the left of the brachiocephalic trunk. The third major branch is the left subclavian artery, which arises posterior and lateral to the left common carotid artery. It is the arterial supply to the majority of the left upper limb.

# Image 2.7

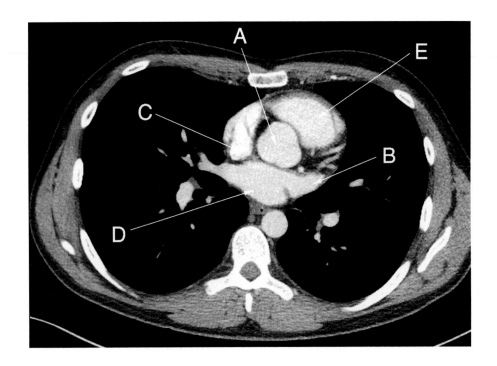

# Image: CT mediastinum axial (2.7)

## ANSWERS

A   Ascending aorta
B   Left atrial appendage
C   Superior vena cava
D   Left atrium
E   Right ventricle/ventricular cavity

## LEARNING POINT

The left atrium is the most posterior of the four cardiac chambers. It receives oxygenated blood from the left and right superior and inferior pulmonary veins. From here the blood is pumped through the mitral valve to the left ventricle.

The left atrium is connected to a finger-like, trabeculated structure called the left atrial appendage. This is located antero-laterally to the main left atrium, arising near the left pulmonary veins.

# Image 2.8

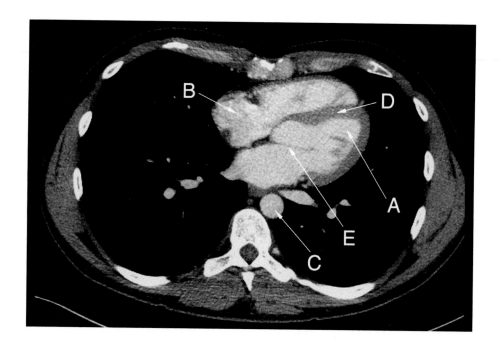

# Image: CT mediastinum axial (2.8)

## ANSWERS

A   Left ventricle/ventricular cavity
B   Right atrium
C   Descending aorta
D   Muscular interventricular septum
E   Mitral valve

## LEARNING POINT

The interventricular septum divides the left ventricle from the right ventricle. It is composed of a muscular part and a membranous part. The muscular part is the larger, longer contribution. The membranous part, which is sited closer to the atria, is the more likely site (90%) for a ventricular septal defect.

# Image 2.9

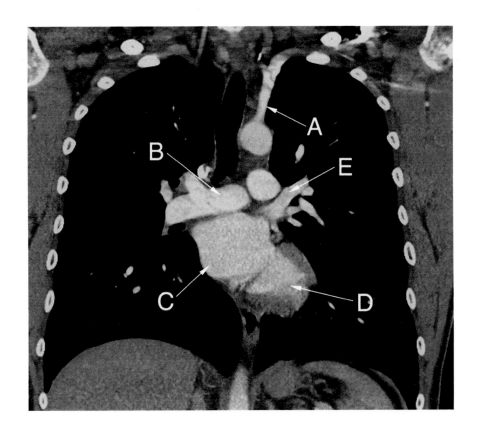

# Image: CT mediastinum coronal (2.9)

## ANSWERS

A   Left subclavian artery
B   Right pulmonary artery
C   Left atrium
D   Left ventricle/ventricular cavity
E   Left superior pulmonary vein

## LEARNING POINT

The left ventricle can be differentiated from the right ventricle by position and morphology. The left ventricle is located posterior to the right ventricle, and has a large contribution to the left heart border. Multi-planar reformats and MR scans can be disorientating at first, but remember that a healthy left ventricle will have a much thicker muscle mass than the right ventricle.

# Image 2.10

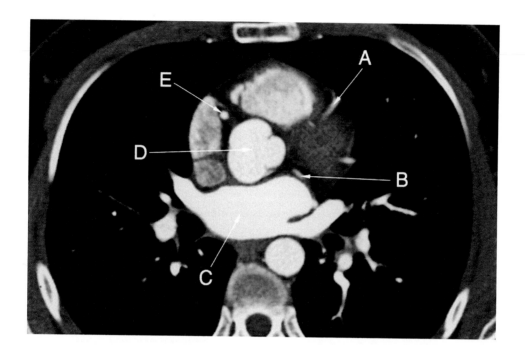

# Image: CT cardiac angiogram (2.10)

## ANSWERS

A   Left anterior descending coronary artery
B   Left circumflex coronary artery
C   Left atrium
D   Aortic root
E   Right main coronary artery

## LEARNING POINT

The aortic root begins distal to the aortic annulus and ends at the sino-tubular junction. The aortic sinuses are small dilatations of the proximal aorta where the coronary arteries arise. There are three sinuses, namely the left, right and posterior (or non-coronary) sinuses.

The right coronary artery originates at the right coronary sinus, and travels in the right atrioventricular groove to the lower margin of the heart, where it turns posteriorly to supply the base of the heart.

The left coronary anatomy is explained on p. 96.

# Image 2.11

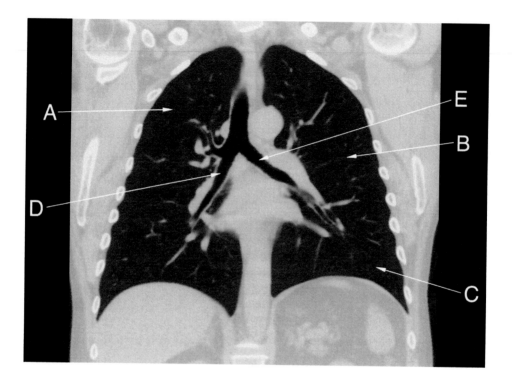

# Image: CT chest coronal (2.11)

## ANSWERS

A   Right upper lobe
B   Left oblique fissure
C   Left lower lobe
D   Bronchus intermedius
E   Left main bronchus

## LEARNING POINT

The trachea divides at the carina into the left and right mainstem bronchi. The right main bronchus is shorter than the left, and is also orientated almost vertically aligned with the trachea. Therefore aspirate or an inhaled foreign body is more likely to obstruct the right main bronchus, or a lobar branch, than the left side.

The bronchus intermedius is the portion of the right bronchial tree distal to the upper lobe bronchus, and before the origin of the middle and lower lobe bronchi.

# Image 2.12

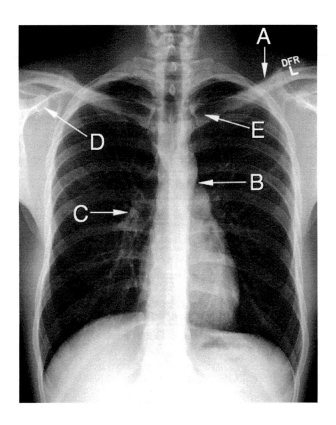

# Image: XR chest PA (2.12)

## ANSWERS

A   Companion shadow
B   Aorto-pulmonary window
C   Right pulmonary artery
D   Right corocoid process
E   Head of left clavicle

## LEARNING POINT

A companion shadow represents a well-defined soft tissue density line seen in parallel to a bony structure. Companion shadows are most commonly seen with regard to the clavicle and the upper ribs, and they are often confused with pathology.

The aorto-pulmonary window is a potential space between the arch of the aorta and the pulmonary artery. A mass within the aorto-pulmonary window may represent an enlarged lymph node.

# Image 2.13

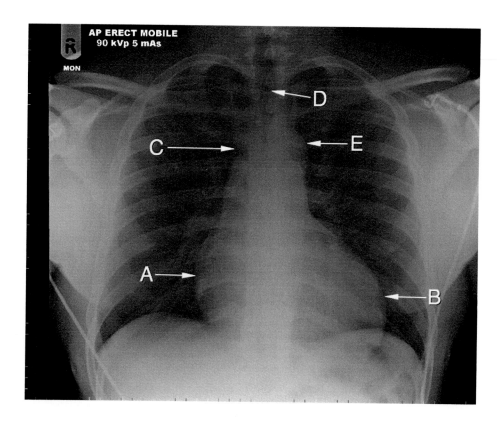

# Image: XR chest PA (2.13)

## ANSWERS

A   Right atrial border
B   Left ventricular border
C   Superior vena cava
D   Trachea
E   Aortic arch

## LEARNING POINT

**Figure 2.13a Diagram line drawing of heart borders.** *See colour plate section.*

# Image 2.14

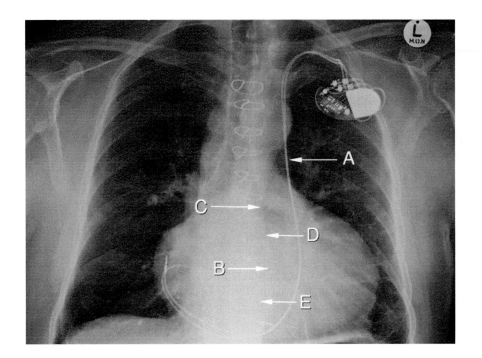

## QUESTIONS

A   Which vessel lies here?
B   Which valve is positioned here?
C   Which valve is positioned here?
D   Which valve is positioned here?
E   Which valve is positioned here?

# Image: XR chest PA with pacemaker (2.14)

## ANSWERS

A   Left-sided superior vena cava
B   Position of mitral valve
C   Position of pulmonary valve
D   Position of aortic valve
E   Position of tricuspid valve

## LEARNING POINT

In this radiograph the pacing wires can clearly be seen to lie on the left-hand side. This patient has bilateral superior vena cavae. This is the most common venous anomaly within the chest, and is seen in approximately 0.5% of the population.

The position of the heart valves runs from superiorly to inferiorly in the following order: pulmonary, aortic, mitral, triscupid.

# Image 2.15

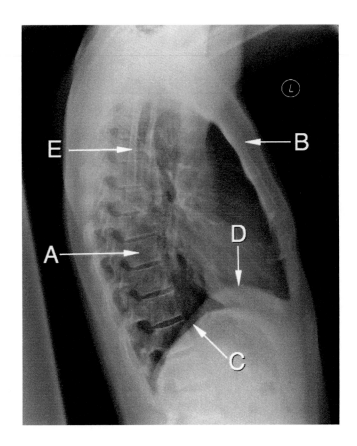

# Image: XR chest lateral (2.15)

## ANSWERS

A   Vertebral body
B   Sternum
C   Left hemidiaphragm
D   Right hemidiaphragm
E   Scapula

## LEARNING POINT

It can be difficult to distinguish the left hemidiaphragm from the right hemidiaphragm on a lateral chest radiograph. The right hemidiaphragm should be visible to the anterior chest wall, but the shadow of the left hemidiaphragm should be lost at the cardiac border.

# Image 2.16

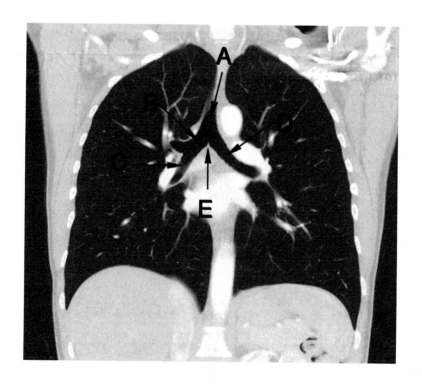

# Image: CT chest coronal (2.16)

## ANSWERS

A   Trachea
B   Right main bronchus
C   Bronchus intermedius
D   Left main bronchus
E   Carina

## LEARNING POINT

The bronchopulmonary segments are as follows:

*Right lung*

Upper lobe
    Anterior segment
    Apical segment
    Posterior segment

Middle lobe
    Medial segment
    Lateral segment

Lower lobe
    Superior segment
    Anterior basal segment
    Medial basal segment
    Lateral basal segment
    Posterior basal segment

*Left lung*

Upper lobe
    Anterior segment
    Apico-posterior segment

Lingula lobe
    Superior segment
    Inferior segment

Lower lobe
    Superior segment
    Anteromedial basal segment

    Lateral basal segment
    Posterior basal segment

**A**lways **A**lways **P**ut **M**iddle **L**obe **S**egments **A**s **M**edial and **L**ateral **P**lease

The above mnemonic can be used to remember the ten lobes on the right, and also to remember that the middle lobe has medial and lateral segments, in comparison with the lingula's superior and inferior segments.

    The left lung has to make space for the heart, and thus the apico-posterior segment is formed from the apical and posterior upper lobe segments, and the anteromedial basal segment is formed from the anterior and medial basal segments.

# Image 2.17

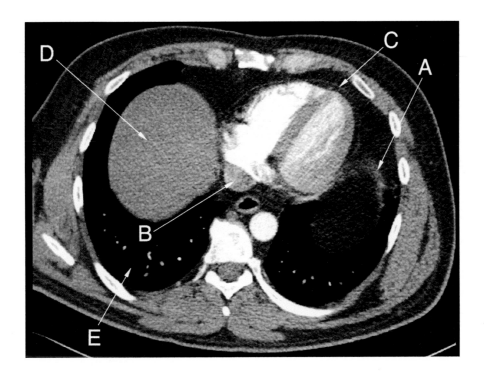

# Image: CT mediastinum axial (2.17)

## ANSWERS

A   Left hemidiaphragm
B   Inferior vena cava
C   Pericardium
D   Right lobe of liver
E   Right lower lobe

## LEARNING POINT

The diaphragm is a complex muscular sheet that separates the thorax from the abdomen. The diaphragm attaches to the costal margin, the xiphoid process, the 11th and 12th ribs, and the second and third lumbar vertebrae.

The diaphragm has a domed appearance, and the superior aspect of the right hemidiaphragm is higher than the left by 1.5 to 2.0 cm, under normal circumstances, in nearly 90% of the population.

# Image 2.18

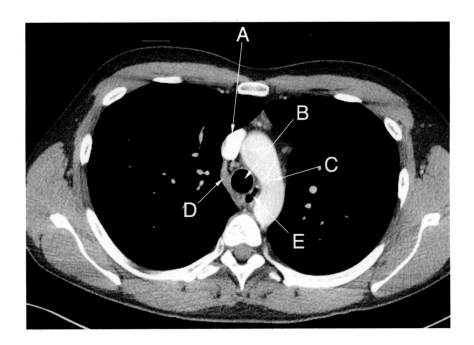

# Image: CT mediastinum axial (2.18)

## ANSWERS

A   Superior vena cava
B   Trachea
C   Aortic arch
D   Azygos arch
E   Oesophagus

## LEARNING POINT

The azygos vein forms part of the azygos system of venous drainage. The azygos vein itself arises on the right side of the first or second lumbar vertebrae and ascends in this position, receiving various tributaries. It runs parallel to the hemiazygos and accessory hemiazygos veins, which ascend and descend on the left side of the thoracic vertebral bodies.

As the azygos vein reaches the root of the right lung, it turns anteriorly to form the azygos arch and then drains into the superior vena cava.

# Image 2.19

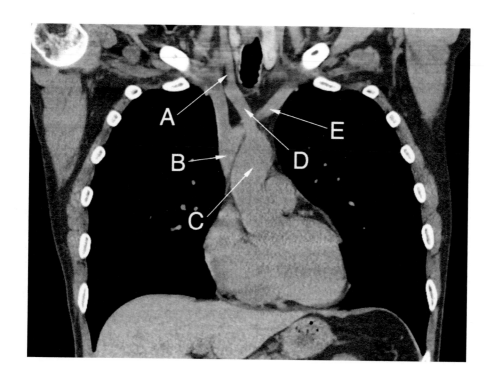

# Image: CT mediastinum coronal (2.19)

## ANSWERS

A  Right common carotid artery
B  Superior vena cava
C  Ascending aorta
D  Brachiocephalic trunk
E  Left brachiocephalic vein

## LEARNING POINT

The vertebral arteries are the first branches of the left and right subclavian arteries as they enter the root of the neck. They pass posteriorly to the ascending common carotid arteries, and therefore are not easily seen on an AP arch angiogram or coronal reconstruction. They then turn further posteriorly to ascend in the foramina transversaria, starting at the C6 level, coursing superiorly to eventually enter the cranial vault through the foramen magnum.

# Image 2.20

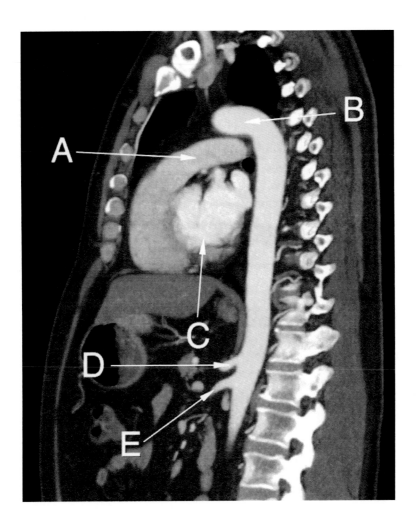

# Image: CT mediastinum sagittal (2.20)

## ANSWERS

A   Pulmonary trunk
B   Aortic arch
C   Left ventricle
D   Coeliac axis
E   Superior mesenteric artery

## LEARNING POINT

When considering the heart and great vessels from a lateral or sagittal point of view, remember the configuration of the pulmonary trunk as it relates to the aorta. The pulmonary trunk lies just to the left of the ascending aorta, and is also shorter than the aorta. Therefore the aorta arches superiorly over the shorter pulmonary trunk, just to the right of its division into the right and left pulmonary arteries. This is the location of the ligamentum arteriosum, embryologically known as the ductus arteriosus, which is the vessel that allows blood to bypass the lungs during fetal development.

# Image 2.21

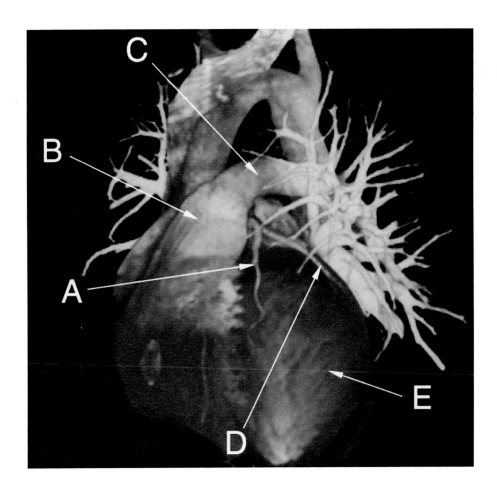

# Image: CT VR heart anterior (2.21)

## ANSWERS

A   Left anterior descending coronary artery
B   Right ventricular outflow tract/pulmonary trunk
C   Main pulmonary artery
D   Left circumflex coronary artery
E   Left ventricle

## LEARNING POINT

The left main coronary artery arises from the left coronary sinus. It passes between the left atrial appendage and pulmonary trunk, and then divides into the left circumflex artery and the left anterior descending artery (LAD). The LAD descends towards the apex of the heart. The left circumflex artery travels in the coronary sulcus, and descends on the posterior surface of the heart heading for the posterior interventricular sulcus.

# Chapter 3
# Chest wall and breast

# Image 3.1

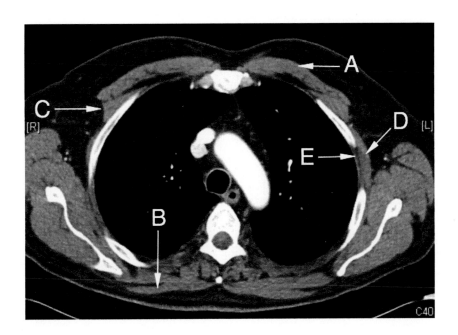

# Image: CT chest axial (3.1)

## ANSWERS

A    Left pectoralis major
B    Right trapezius
C    Right pectoralis minor
D    Left serratus anterior
E    Left intercostal muscle

## LEARNING POINT

Most of the 'chest wall' muscles are strictly shoulder muscles, but as they are visible on a chest CT we have included them here. They should be easy to recognise. The pectoralis muscles lie on the anterior aspect of the chest wall, with the major lying on top of the minor. The serratus anterior attaches the medial aspect of the scapula to the upper eight or nine ribs.

The intercostal muscles are true chest wall muscles and are involved in respiration. It is important to remember that they are made of three components, namely the external intercostal, internal intercostal and innermost intercostal groups. The neurovascular bundle sits between the internal and innermost segments. It is positioned in a groove lying inferiorly in the rib. When marking, tapping or draining chests it is best to avoid the neurovascular bundle by aiming immediately above the rib.

# Image 3.2

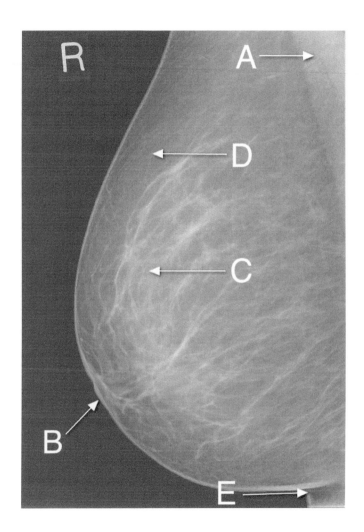

# Image: XR mammogram MLO (3.2)

## ANSWERS

A   Pectoralis major
B   Nipple
C   Glandular tissue
D   Adipose tissue
E   Inframammary fold

## LEARNING POINT

This is a mediolateral oblique (MLO) view. It is one of two standard views used routinely in mammography. The aim of the MLO view is to achieve visible pectoralis major muscle to at least the level of the nipple, and to demonstrate the inframammary fold. Lymph nodes are often visible towards the top of the film as the image extends into the axilla.

   The other standard view is a craniocaudal (CC) view. This view contains the pectoral muscle posteriorly, and should demonstrate the nipple in profile. The position of the nipple can help to determine the position of a mass. If lateral to the nipple this means that it is in the outer half, and if medial to the nipple it is in the inner half.

# Image 3.3

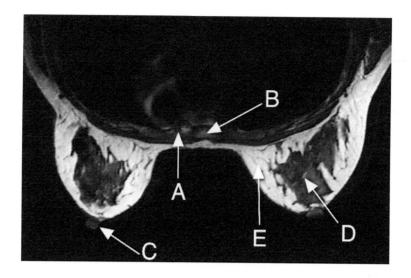

# Image: MR mammogram axial/ CC (3.3)

## ANSWERS

A   Internal thoracic vessels
B   Sternum
C   Nipple
D   Fibroglandular tissue
E   Adipose tissue

## LEARNING POINT

MRI mammography is used to provide additional information to mammographic findings. MRI clearly gives good soft tissue demonstration, but post-contrast tissue enhancement kinetics are also being used to help to assess malignancy.

The internal thoracic vessels run posterior to the intercostal muscles. They can be found lateral to the sternum but medial to the nipple. They are continuous with the superior epigastric vessels. The vein drains into the brachiocephalic vein and the artery arises from the subclavian artery.

# Chapter 4
# Gastrointestinal

# Image 4.1

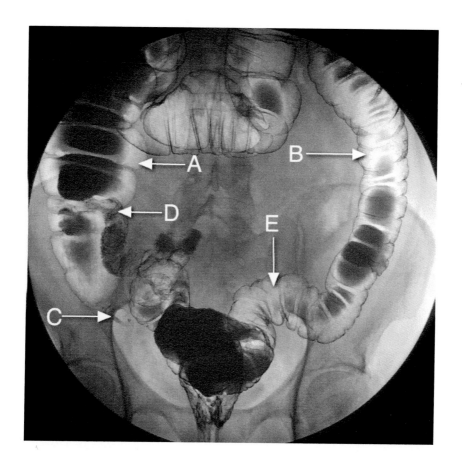

# Image: XR double-contrast barium enema (4.1)

## ANSWERS

A   Ascending colon
B   Descending colon
C   Appendix
D   Terminal ileum
E   Sigmoid colon

## LEARNING POINT

The colonic segments are named with respect to the direction of peristalsis. The ascending colon is the right-sided portion commencing from the caecum. The ascending colon becomes the transverse colon at the hepatic flexure and continues to the splenic flexure. The descending colon runs on the left side of the abdomen from the splenic flexure to the sigmoid colon.

The appendix is a variable structure. It varies in length and also in the position of its tip. However, the origin is fairly consistently found at the posteromedial aspect of the caecum. It measures approximately 10 cm in length, and the tip may be seen in several different positions. Most commonly the tip may be retrocaecal, pelvic or extraperitoneal.

# Image 4.2

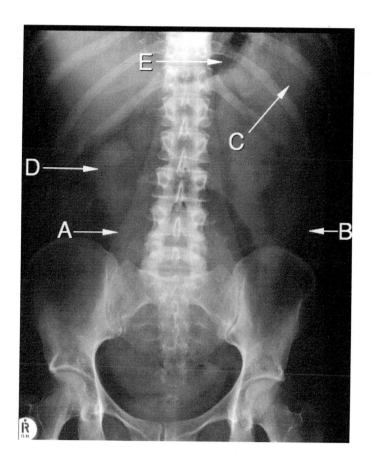

# Image: XR abdomen AP (4.2)

## ANSWERS

A  Right psoas shadow
B  Left properitoneal line
C  Spleen
D  Right kidney
E  Stomach

## LEARNING POINT

The properitoneal line or fat stripe is formed from a layer of fat between the parietal peritoneum and the abdominal wall. On a radiograph the properitoneal line is seen between the abdominal muscles and the colon. It may become blurred in acute appendicitis or increased with ascites.

# Image 4.3

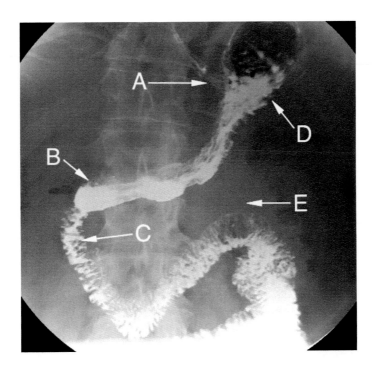

## QUESTIONS

A   Name the structure labelled A.
B   Name the structure labelled B.
C   Name the structure labelled C.
D   Name the structure labelled D.
E   Which ligament lies at this point?

# Image: XR barium meal (4.3)

## ANSWERS

A   Oesophagus
B   First part of duodenum
C   Second part of duodenum
D   Greater curve of stomach
E   Ligament of Treitz

## LEARNING POINT

The duodenum is the first part of the small bowel, and it commences at the pylorus with the duodenal bulb or cap. The first part courses right and then turns inferiorly at the superior duodenal flexure. This vertical segment becomes the second part of the duodenum. This contains the ampulla of Vater, which delineates the junction of the embryological foregut and midgut. The second part of the duodenum ends after it has turned left to become horizontal again. The third part is essentially the horizontal section that crosses the midline. The fourth part passes superiorly to the duodenojejunal flexure at the ligament of Treitz. The ligament of Treitz is a fixed point that marks the transition from duodenum to jejunum.

# Image 4.4

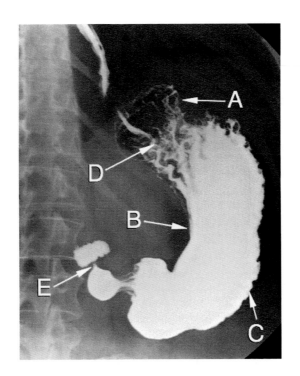

# Image: XR barium meal (4.4)

## ANSWERS

A   Fundus of stomach
B   Lesser curve of stomach
C   Greater curve of stomach
D   Gastro-oesophageal junction
E   Pylorus

## LEARNING POINT

The radiological anatomy of the stomach is fairly simple. The long lateral border is termed the greater curve and shorter medial border is termed the lesser curve. Between the two curves is the body of the stomach. The fundus is at the top and the pylorus is at the bottom. The gastro-oesophageal junction is often termed the cardia.

    The stomach receives its blood supply from branches of the coeliac axis. The left gastric artery branches from the coeliac axis directly and supplies the superior portion of the lesser curve. The right gastric artery supplies the inferior portion of the lesser curve, which is a branch of the common hepatic. The left and right gastroepiploic arteries supply the greater curve. Once again the left gastroepiploic artery supplies the superior portion, and the right gastroepiploic artery supplies the inferior portion. The left is a branch of the splenic artery and the right is a branch of the gastroduodenal artery. The fundus is supplied by the short gastric arteries arising from the splenic artery.

    Remember, left superior, rIght Inferior.

# Image 4.5

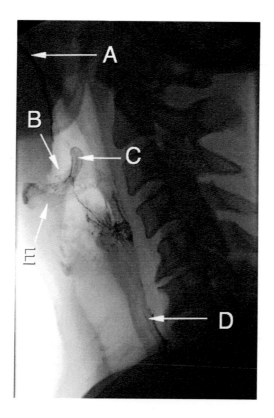

# Image: XR contrast swallow pharynx lateral (4.5)

## ANSWERS

A   Base of tongue
B   Vallecula
C   Epiglottis
D   Oesophagus
E   Hyoid bone

## LEARNING POINT

The pharynx refers to anything between the nasal cavity and the larynx. It is subdivided into three sections:

- nasopharynx – skull base to soft palate
- oropharynx – soft palate to hyoid bone
- hypopharynx – hyoid bone to cricopharyngeus muscle.

# Image 4.6

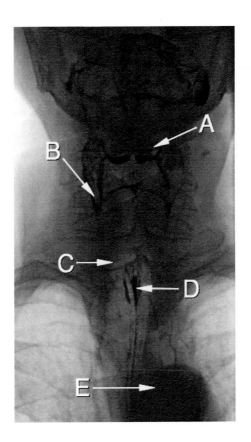

# Image: Contrast swallow pharynx AP (4.6)

## ANSWERS

A  Left vallecula
B  Right piriform fossa
C  Trachea
D  Oesophagus
E  Aortic arch

## LEARNING POINT

In the presence of a dysfunctional swallow, portions of the swallowed bolus may pool in the valleculae or the piriform fossae. If this does not initially result in clinically apparent aspiration, it may become noticeable following subsequent boluses. As the valleculae or piriform fossae become full they will spill over and lead to penetration and/or aspiration.

# Image 4.7

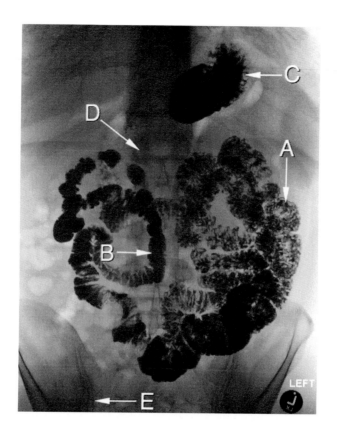

# Image: XR barium follow through (4.7)

## ANSWERS

A  Jejunum
B  Ileum
C  Stomach
D  Pedicle of L1
E  Right sacroiliac joint

## LEARNING POINT

It can be difficult to distinguish the different parts of small bowel on contrast studies and CT. The following features help to identify them:

|  | Jejunum | Ileum |
|---|---|---|
| Site | Proximal | Distal |
| Lumen | Wider | Smaller |
| Valvulae conniventes | Prominent | Thinner and fewer |
| Wall | Thick | Thin |
| Mucosa | Featured | Featureless |

# Image 4.8

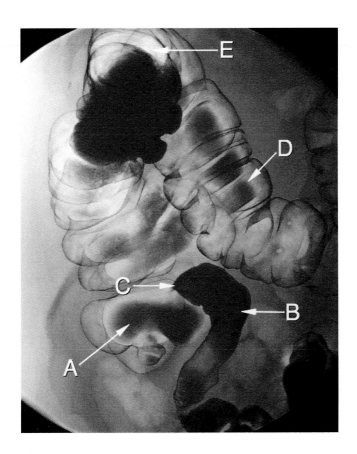

# Image: XR contrast study (4.8)

## ANSWERS

A  Caecum
B  Terminal ileum
C  Ileocaecal valve
D  Transverse colon
E  Hepatic flexure

## LEARNING POINT

The caecum represents the beginning of the large bowel. It is usually situated in the right iliac fossa. Caecal volvulus causes large bowel obstruction and is usually diagnosed on abdominal radiograph. Two forms are recognised, namely true volvulus and bascule.

True volvulus is caused by axial torsion. The caecum twists along the long axis of the ascending colon. A dilated caecum may be seen to extend from the right iliac fossa to the left upper quadrant. The distal large bowel is commonly decompressed, and the proximal small bowel is dilated.

Caecal bascule refers to the caecum folding upwards and medially towards the ascending colon. This tends to give rise to a centrally positioned dilated caecum, and the small bowel may often look normal.

# Image 4.9

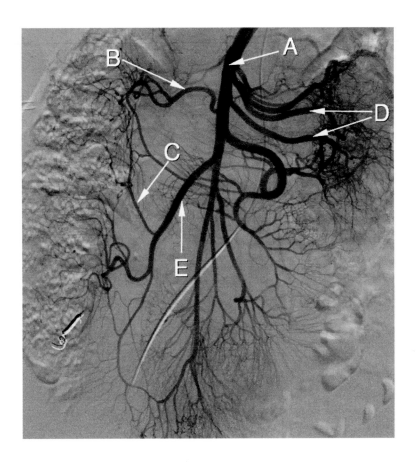

# Image: DSA superior mesenteric artery (4.9)

## ANSWERS

A   Superior mesenteric artery
B   Middle colic artery
C   Right colic artery
D   Jejunal branches of superior mesenteric artery
E   Ileo-colic artery

## LEARNING POINT

The blood supply to the gut is determined by the embryological development of the gut. The gut is divided embryologically into the foregut, midgut and hindgut. The three main arteries supplying the gut are the coeliac axis, the superior mesenteric artery and the inferior mesenteric artery. The foregut is supplied by the coeliac axis, the midgut by the superior mesenteric artery, and the hindgut by the inferior mesenteric artery.

The blood supply can be summarised as follows:

Coeliac axis
    Foregut
        Abdominal oesophagus
        Stomach
        First and second parts of duodenum

Superior mesenteric artery
    Midgut
        Third and fourth parts of duodenum
        Jejunum
        Ileum
        Caecum
        Ascending colon
        Proximal two-thirds of transverse colon

Inferior mesenteric artery
    Hindgut
        Distal third of transverse colon
        Descending colon
        Sigmoid colon
        Rectum

# Image 4.10

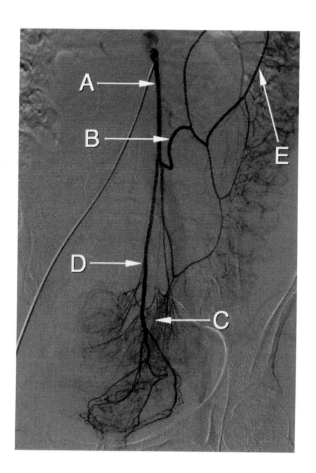

# Image: DSA inferior mesenteric artery (4.10)

## ANSWERS

A  Inferior mesenteric artery
B  Left colic artery
C  Sigmoid branches of inferior mesenteric artery
D  Superior rectal branch of inferior mesenteric artery
E  Marginal artery of Drummond

## LEARNING POINT

The inferior mesenteric artery is the primary blood supply to the descending colon, the sigmoid colon and the superior part of the rectum. The branches are named after the area of supply. The marginal artery forms an anastomosis between the inferior and superior mesenteric arteries and supplies the splenic flexure. The splenic flexure is a 'watershed area' and is thus vulnerable to ischaemia.

# Chapter 5
# Upper abdominal viscera

# Image 5.1

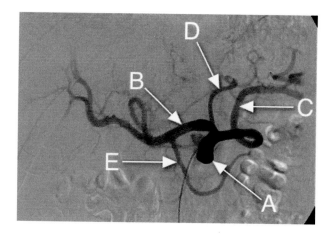

# Image: DSA coeliac axis (5.1)

## ANSWERS

A  Coeliac trunk
B  Common hepatic artery
C  Splenic artery
D  Left gastric artery
E  Gastroduodenal artery

## LEARNING POINT

The coeliac trunk arises from the abdominal aorta at the level of T12 and supplies the organs of the embryological foregut. These organs consist of the liver, the spleen, the stomach, the abdominal oesophagus, the superior portion of the pancreas, and the first and second parts of the duodenum.

The anatomy demonstrated here is the conventional anatomy. However, it should be noted that there are many variants, and classical anatomy may be seen in as few as 50% of patients.

# Image 5.2

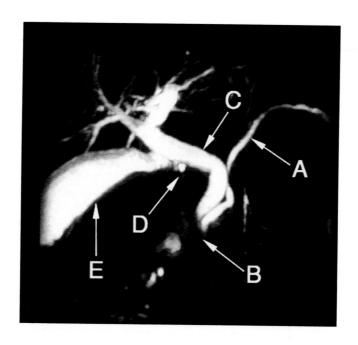

# Image: Magnetic resonance cholangiopancreatogram (5.2)

## ANSWERS

A   Main pancreatic duct
B   Ampulla of Vater
C   Common bile duct
D   Cystic duct
E   Gallbladder

## LEARNING POINT

The conventional anatomy of the pancreatic ducts is for the main pancreatic duct and the common bile duct to merge at the ampulla of Vater. The ampulla is a solitary opening into the duodenum. In approximately 5% of the population there are separate openings for both the main pancreatic duct and the common bile duct. A third variant affects approximately 10% of the population and is termed pancreas divisum. Here the dorsal and ventral parts of the pancreas fail to fuse and as such the main pancreatic drainage is through the duct of Santorini. The common bile duct and the ventral duct use the ampulla of Vater.

Normal

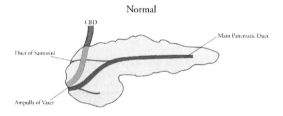

Separate Openings

Pancreas Divisum

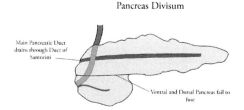

**Figure 5.2a Diagram of pancreatic variations. *Please refer to the colour version in the plate section.***

# Image 5.3

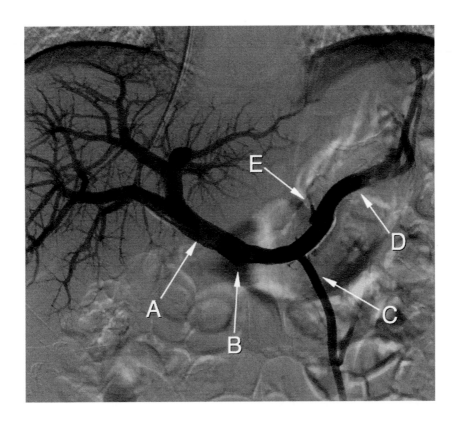

# Image: Direct portal venogram (5.3)

## ANSWERS

A   Portal vein
B   Superior mesenteric vein insertion
C   Inferior mesenteric vein
D   Splenic vein
E   Left gastric vein

## LEARNING POINT

The portal vein receives blood from three major branches, namely the inferior mesenteric vein, the superior mesenteric vein and the splenic vein. The inferior mesenteric vein usually drains directly into the splenic vein behind the body or tail of the pancreas. The superior mesenteric vein joins the portal system posterior to the neck of the pancreas. The common anatomical variations of the portal venous system include the inferior mesenteric vein anastomosing with the superior mesenteric vein directly, or the inferior mesenteric vein draining into the confluence of the splenic vein and the superior mesenteric vein.

# Image 5.4

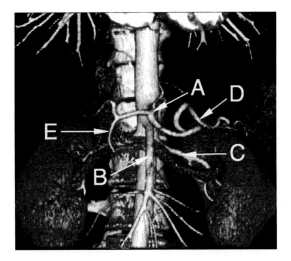

*Please refer to the colour version in the plate section.*

# Image: CT aortogram vascular reconstruction (5.4)

## ANSWERS

A   Coeliac trunk
B   Superior mesenteric artery
C   Left renal artery
D   Splenic artery
E   Gastroduodenal artery

## LEARNING POINT

The order of the visceral branches of the abdominal aorta may be remembered using the following mnemonic:

**C**ancer **S**taging **M**eans **R**adiologists **G**et **I**nvolved

**C**oeliac axis
**S**uperior mesenteric
**M**iddle suprarenal
**R**enal
**G**onadal
**I**nferior mesenteric

It is important to remember that there are two sets of parietal arteries, namely the inferior phrenic arteries and four paired lumbar arteries.

# Image 5.5

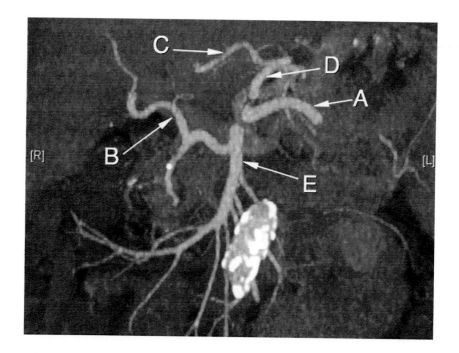

# Image: MIP of abdominal vasculature (5.5)

## ANSWERS

A  Splenic artery
B  Right hepatic artery
C  Left hepatic artery
D  Left gastric artery
E  Superior mesenteric artery

## LEARNING POINT

This image demonstrates an anatomical variation, in this case a replaced right hepatic artery. The right hepatic artery arises from the superior mesenteric artery. There is a contribution to the hepatic supply from the coeliac trunk via the left hepatic artery. In approximately 20% of the population all or part of their hepatic supply arises from a replaced or accessory vessel from the superior mesenteric artery.

    This image may seem confusing at first. If you cannot immediately identify the anatomy, start from first principles. We know that the coeliac axis should give three vessels – the splenic, left gastric and common hepatic arteries. We know the classical shape of the superior mesenteric artery. In this image the superior mesenteric artery (E), the splenic artery (A) and the left gastric artery (D) are easily identified. By a process of elimination the other vessels (B and C) must be the hepatic arteries.

# Image 5.6

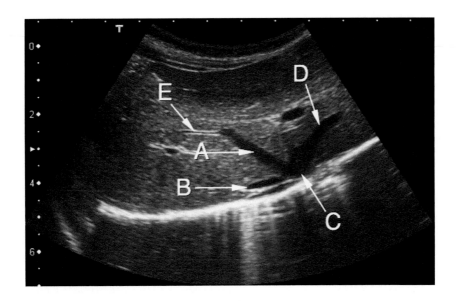

# Image: US liver transverse (5.6)

## ANSWERS

A   Middle hepatic vein
B   Right hepatic vein
C   Inferior vena cava
D   Left hepatic vein
E   Portal vein branch/intrahepatic biliary duct

## LEARNING POINT

The liver is divided into functional segments by the Couinaud classification. The liver is split into superior and inferior halves by the portal vein. The hepatic veins further divide the liver into segments in a sagittal plane. This gives rise to the eight functional liver segments. The caudate is segment 1, and the remainder are numbered in a clockwise manner. Remember that segment 4 is often divided into 4a superiorly and 4b inferiorly.

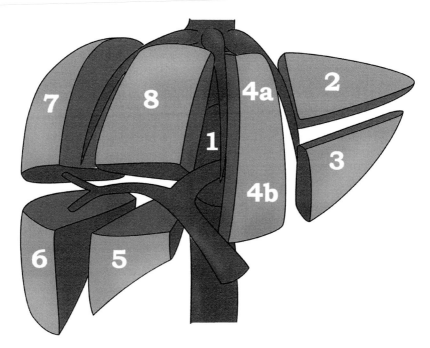

**Figure 5.6a Diagram of liver segments.** *Please refer to the colour version in the plate section.*

# Image 5.7

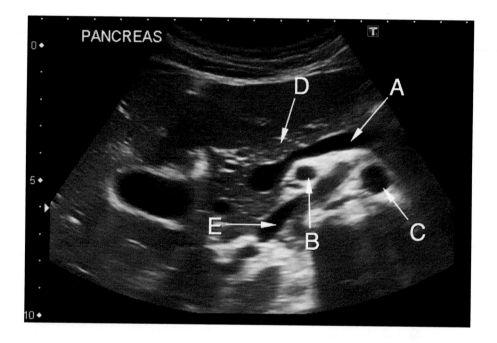

# Image: US pancreas transverse (5.7)

## ANSWERS

A   Splenic vein
B   Superior mesenteric artery
C   Abdominal aorta
D   Neck of pancreas
E   Inferior vena cava

## LEARNING POINT

This is a standard transverse abdominal ultrasound view. Underneath the left lobe of the liver are the body and tail of the pancreas. As previously described, the splenic vein passes from left to right behind the pancreas to converge with the inferior mesenteric vein and then the superior mesenteric vein to form the portal vein. The superior mesenteric artery can be seen arching anteriorly from the aorta over the left renal vein but under the splenic vein.

# Image 5.8

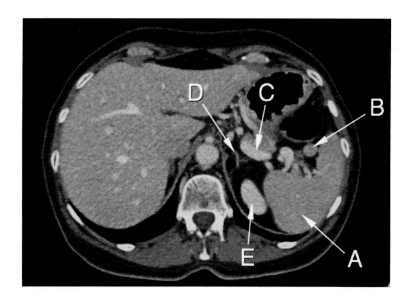

# Image: CT abdomen axial (5.8)

## ANSWERS

A    Spleen
B    Splenunculus
C    Splenic artery
D    Left adrenal gland
E    Left kidney

## LEARNING POINT

The presence of a splenunculus is a common and benign finding. It is important to confirm it as accessory splenic tissue and distinguish it from other pathology such as a lymph node or peritoneal metastasis. On CT a splenunculus should be in close proximity to the spleen, round in shape, and share the same attenuation characteristics as the spleen. Splenunculi are different from splenosis. The latter refers to abdominal splenic tissue that is deposited following abdominal trauma or splenectomy. Splenunculi have a splenic blood supply, whereas splenosis does not.

# Image 5.9

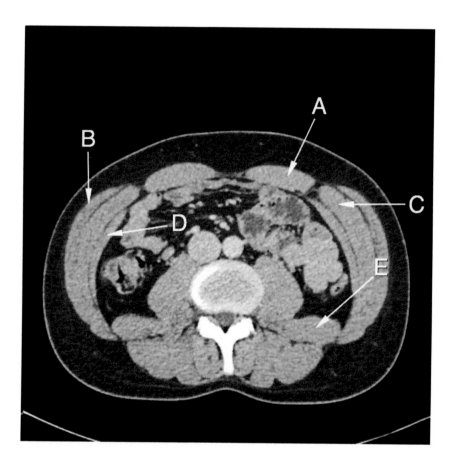

# Image: CT abdomen axial (5.9)

## ANSWERS

A   Left rectus abdominis
B   Right external oblique
C   Left internal oblique
D   Right transversus abdominis
E   Left quadratus lumborum

## LEARNING POINT

Identifying the abdominal wall muscles should be routine. The anterior abdominal wall muscles are the rectus abdominis muscles, separated by the linea alba.

The three lateral wall muscles are only slightly more complex. The external oblique is the most superficial, with the internal oblique beneath it. The innermost muscle is the transversus abdominis.

# Image 5.10

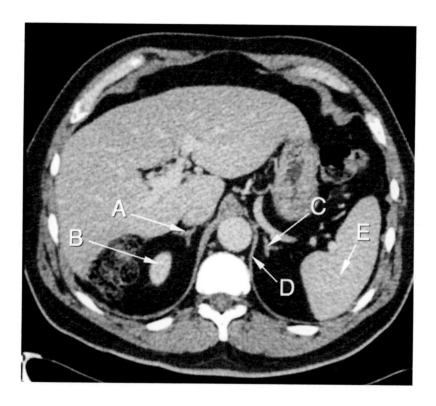

# Image: CT abdomen axial (5.10)

## ANSWERS

A   Right adrenal gland
B   Right kidney
C   Left adrenal gland
D   Crus of left diaphragm
E   Spleen

## LEARNING POINT

Normal adrenal glands can be a challenge to identify. They are small and often squashed. They sit within the perirenal fat superior to the kidneys and lateral to the diaphragmatic crura.

The classical appearance of the adrenal gland is that of a tricorn hat or an inverted Y. Essentially there are two limbs converging on the body anteriorly.

# Image 5.11

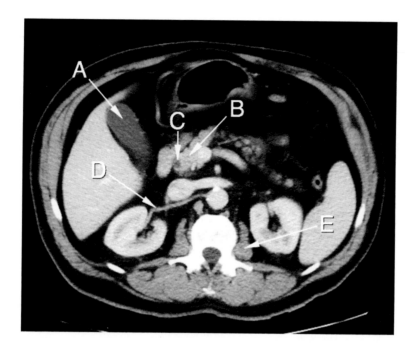

# Image: CT abdomen axial (5.11)

## ANSWERS

A   Gallbladder
B   Head of pancreas
C   Common bile duct
D   Right renal artery
E   Left psoas

## LEARNING POINT

Although it is not usually the primary method of investigating biliary disease, CT does allow visualisation of the common bile duct as it enters the pancreatic head. The normal diameter of the common bile duct is 6–7 mm. This may be enlarged following cholecystectomy or in an ageing patient without having a pathological cause.

# Image 5.12

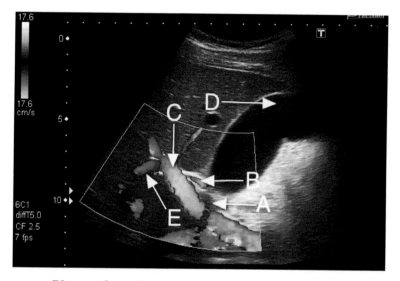

*Please refer to the colour version in the plate section.*

# Image: USS porta hepatis (5.12)

## ANSWERS

A   Common bile duct
B   Hepatic artery
C   Portal vein
D   Gallbladder
E   Hepatic vein

## LEARNING POINT

Ultrasound is usually the first examination in assessment of the biliary tree. When searching for the common bile duct it is often easier to first identify the portal vein in the porta hepatis and then try to find the duct. The duct should be anterior to the portal vein and the hepatic artery. Another useful distinguishing feature is that the duct should be straight, whereas the artery commonly takes a tortuous route. Of course the artery should have flow whereas the common bile duct should not.

# Image 5.13

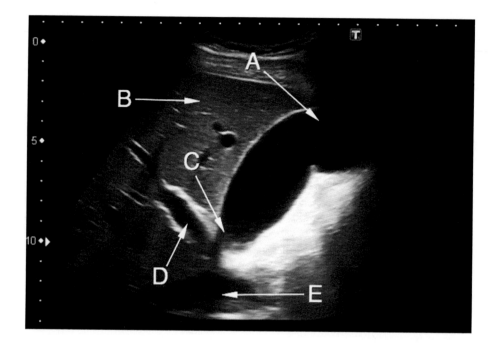

# Image: USS gallbladder (5.13)

## ANSWERS

A   Fundus of gallbladder
B   Liver
C   Neck of gallbladder
D   Portal vein
E   Inferior vena cava

## LEARNING POINT

Assessment of the gallbladder is commonly performed using ultrasound. The gallbladder is classically found on the inferior surface of the liver at the junction of the two lobes. This position is variable, but a distended gallbladder can usually be identified. The gallbladder consists of a fundus distally, a body, and a neck proximally as it tapers into the cystic duct. The most common variation in shape is the 'Phrygian cap'. This normal variant describes the folding of the gallbladder fundus over the body. The normal gallbladder wall thickness is less than 3 mm.

# Image 5.14

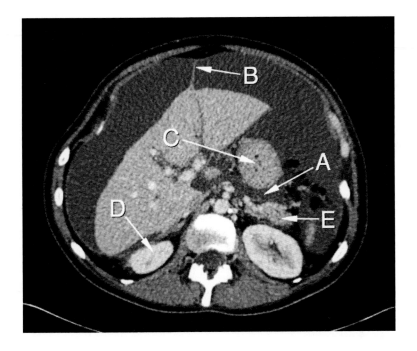

# Image: CT upper abdomen (5.14)

## ANSWERS

A  Lesser sac
B  Falciform ligament
C  Stomach
D  Right kidney
E  Tail of pancreas

## LEARNING POINT

The lesser sac is a potential space between the posterior aspect of the stomach and the pancreas. The lesser sac communicates through the foramen of Winslow (or epiploic foramen) with the rest of the peritoneal cavity (also termed the greater sac). In this image the lesser sac is visible due to ascites in the abdomen.

# Chapter 6
# Genitourinary

## Image 6.1

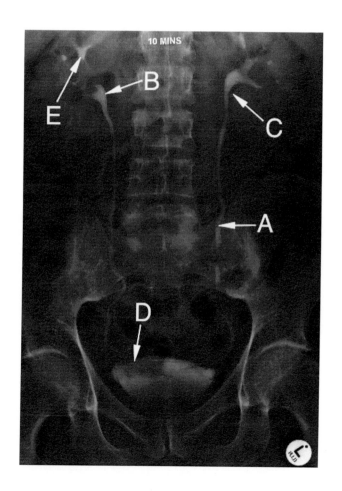

# Image: XR intravenous urogram (6.1)

## ANSWERS

A   Left ureter
B   Right renal pelvis
C   Left pelviureteric junction
D   Right vesicoureteric junction
E   Right upper pole calyx

## LEARNING POINT

The normal anatomy seen on an intravenous urogram consists of the following. The renal calyces drain into the renal pelvis. The renal pelvis becomes the ureter at the pelviureteric junction (PUJ). The ureter continues retroperitoneally to insert into the trigone of the bladder at the vesicoureteric junction (VUJ).

Common variations exist throughout the urinary tract. There are variations in renal form, renal number and renal position, and also variations in ureteric number, ureteric form and ureteric position. Whatever the variation may be, the basic anatomical principles still apply. There will usually still be renal calyces, a renal pelvis, a PUJ, a ureter and a VUJ.

# Image 6.2

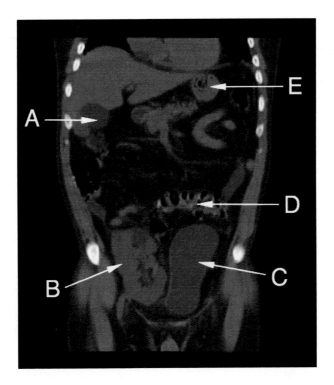

# Image: CT pelvic kidney (6.2)

## ANSWERS

A   Gallbladder
B   Pelvic kidney
C   Bladder
D   Sigmoid colon
E   Stomach

## LEARNING POINT

The two possible causes of an abnormally placed kidney are congenital (renal ectopia) and surgical (transplant). Renal ectopia occurs in approximately 1 in 1000 births and describes a kidney that has failed to take up its normal position. The fetal kidney develops in the pelvis and then rises to its standard position during development. Failure to complete this journey may result in a pelvic kidney, or even in fusion with the contralateral kidney, as in crossed renal ectopia.

This image demonstrates a transplanted kidney. Understanding the anatomy is crucial when assessing a transplanted kidney. The standard surgical procedure is to transplant a left kidney into the right iliac fossa, or a right kidney into the left iliac fossa. Each kidney is turned back to front (i.e. posterior becomes anterior), as if being folded across the midline of the abdomen. The external iliac vessels are preferred for the vascular anastomosis, and the ureter is connected to the dome of the bladder. It is important to remember that with the new orientation of the kidney, the ureter is now anterior to the vessels.

# Image 6.3

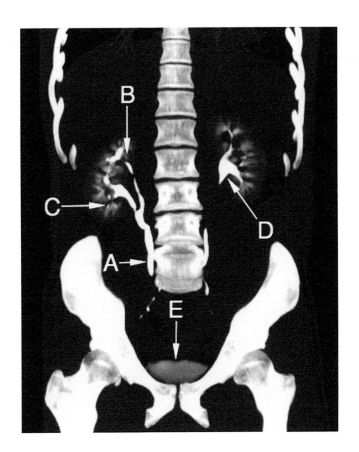

# Image: CT urogram (6.3)

## ANSWERS

A  Right ureter
B  Upper pole moiety of right kidney
C  Lower pole moiety of right kidney
D  Left renal pelvis
E  Urinary bladder

## LEARNING POINT

Ureteric duplication is a common anatomical variation. It may represent duplication of the entire ureter (complete duplication) or a portion of the ureter with convergence of the duplex system at a point along the length of the ureter (incomplete duplication). Duplication is seen in approximately 0.5% of the population. Ureteric duplication is usually an incidental finding and of little clinical significance. However, there may be an increased incidence of reflux, infection and obstruction.

# Image 6.4

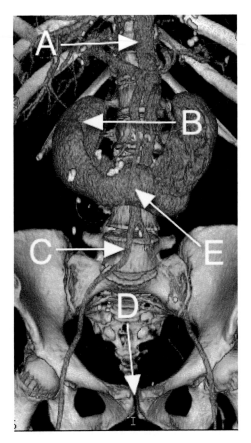

*Please refer to the colour version in the plate section.*

# Image: CT abdomen VR – horseshoe kidney (6.4)

## ANSWERS

A   Aorta
B   Right kidney
C   Right common iliac artery
D   Pubic symphysis
E   Isthmus of horseshoe

## LEARNING POINT

The horseshoe kidney is a congenital fusion variant and affects approximately 1 in 400 of the population. The fusion commonly occurs at the lower poles and causes a degree of malrotation. Although this may be an incidental finding, a horseshoe kidney is associated with increased infection rates, increased stone formation rates, and trauma to the isthmus crossing the midline.

# Image 6.5

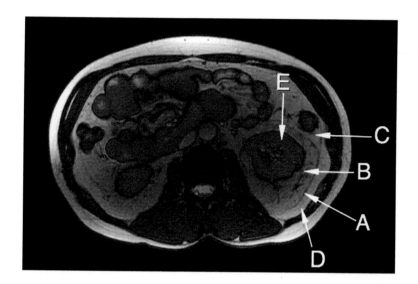

# Image: MR kidneys axial (6.5)

## ANSWERS

A  Perirenal fascia
B  Perirenal fat
C  Anterior pararenal space
D  Posterior pararenal space
E  Left kidney

## LEARNING POINT

The retroperitoneal space is usually divided into three sections, namely the perirenal space (PS), the anterior pararenal space (APS) and the posterior pararenal space (PPS). The perirenal space surrounds the kidney and is enclosed by the perirenal fascia. The perirenal space contains the kidney, adrenal gland, proximal ureter and perirenal fat. The perirenal fascia is traditionally divided into two parts. The anterior reflection is called Gerota's fascia and the posterior reflection is called Zuckerkandl's fascia. Between Gerota's fascia and the parietal peritoneum is the anterior pararenal space, which contains the pancreas, the duodenum and the retroperitoneal sections of ascending and descending colon. The posterior pararenal space is between Zuckerkandl's fascia and the transversalis fascia posteriorly. There are no major organs within the posterior pararenal space, only vessels, fat and lymphatics.

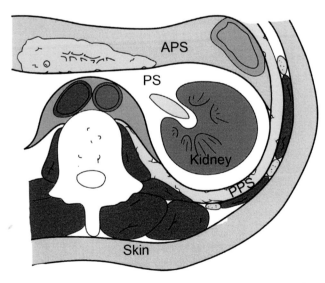

**Figure 6.5a Diagram of fascial trifurcation.** *Please refer to the colour version in the plate section.*

# Image 6.6

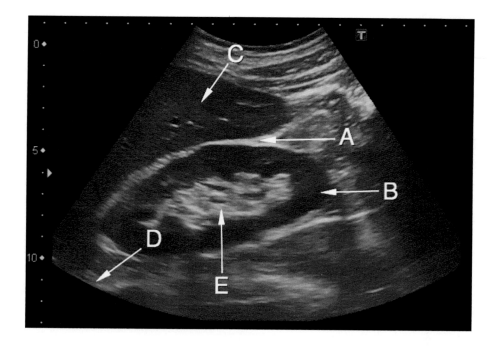

# Image: US right kidney (6.6)

## ANSWERS

A   Morrison's pouch (hepatorenal recess)
B   Lower pole of right kidney
C   Right lobe of liver
D   Right hemidiaphragm
E   Renal sinus fat

## LEARNING POINT

Morrison's pouch is also called the hepatorenal recess and is a potential space. It separates the right kidney from the right lobe of the liver, and in normal conditions is seen only as an interface between the two structures. Intraperitoneal fluid may accumulate within Morrison's pouch, and should be easily visualised with ultrasound.

# Image 6.7

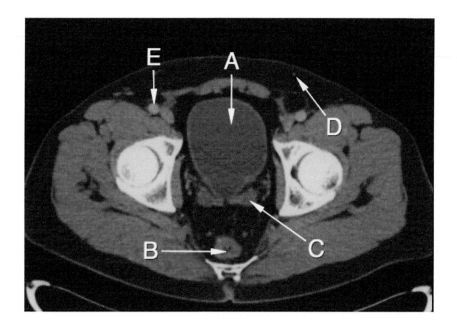

# Image: CT male pelvis (6.7)

## ANSWERS

A   Bladder
B   Rectum
C   Left seminal vesicle
D   Left inferior epigastric vessel
E   Right femoral artery

## LEARNING POINT

The seminal vesicles are paired structures that are approximately 5 cm in diameter. They sit on top of the prostate gland and somewhat resemble a rabbit's ears. They store fluid that is excreted in the ejaculate. The seminal vesicle opens into the vas deferens as it enters the prostate gland. The vasa are also paired structures. However, they arise from the epididymis and travel within the spermatic cord to enter the prostate as the ampullae. Each ampulla is medial to its seminal vesicle.

# Image 6.8

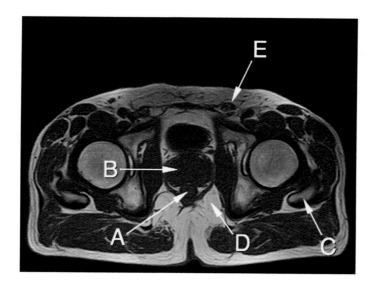

# Image: MR male pelvis axial (6.8)

## ANSWERS

A   Rectum
B   Prostate
C   Left greater trochanter
D   Left ischioanal fossa
E   Left spermatic cord

## LEARNING POINT

Assessment of the prostate gland by MRI is usually reserved for the local staging of prostatic cancer. This image clearly demonstrates the proximity of the prostate to the rectum. This proximity makes assessment and biopsy of the prostate via transrectal ultrasound possible.

The prostate gland is divided into three zones. The central zone sits at the base of the prostate, and this is where the ducts and vasa enter. The transitional zone surrounds the urethra and enlarges in benign prostatic hypertrophy. The peripheral zone is the site of most prostate cancers. The peripheral zone encases the gland rather like a hand cupping a ball.

# Image 6.9

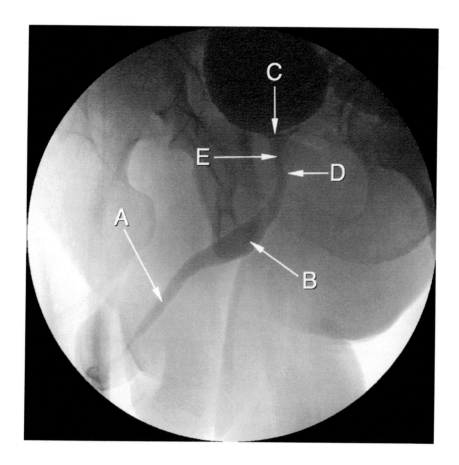

# Image: Male urethrogram (6.9)

## ANSWERS

A  Penile urethra
B  Bulbous urethra
C  Bladder neck
D  External sphincter
E  Position of verumontanum

## LEARNING POINT

A retrograde urethrogram is often performed if there is an indication or suspicion of urethral trauma. Straddle injuries most commonly affect the bulbous urethra, whereas pelvic fractures tend to disrupt the junction of the membranous and prostatic urethra.

The urethra begins with the prostatic urethra proximally. It incorporates the verumontanum prior to reaching the external sphincter that surrounds the short membranous urethra. Distal to the membranous urethra is the larger-calibre bulbous urethra. Finally, the penile urethra extends to the urethral meatus and is of variable length.

# Image 6.10

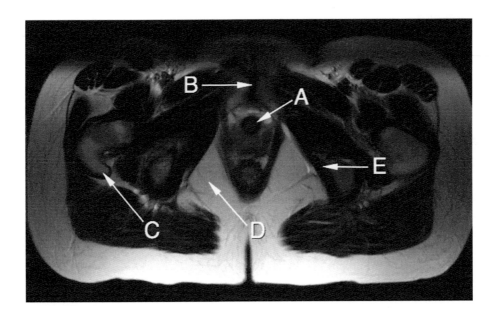

# Image: MR female pelvis (6.10)

## ANSWERS

| | |
|---|---|
| A | Urethra |
| B | Pubic symphysis |
| C | Right greater trochanter |
| D | Right ischioanal fossa |
| E | Left obturator internus |

## LEARNING POINT

The female urethra is clearly shorter than the male urethra. It measures approximately 4 cm and is embedded within the anterior vaginal wall. It courses antero-inferiorly from the bladder to the external meatus. The external urethral meatus is found between the clitoris and the vagina. Radiological investigation and examination of the female urethra is not routine. Fortunately, urethral injuries are less common in females than in males, and therefore urethrography is rarely performed. Transperineal and transvaginal ultrasonography can be performed, and also MRI.

# Image 6.11

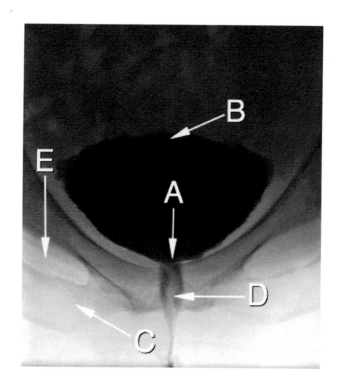

# Image: Cystogram (6.11)

## ANSWERS

A   Bladder neck
B   Bladder fundus
C   Right inferior pubic ramus
D   Urethra
E   Right obturator foramen

## LEARNING POINT

The shape and appearance of the urinary bladder vary with age and also with bladder distension. The bladder of a young child sits higher in the abdomen than that of an adult. An empty bladder collapses down towards the bladder neck and looks like an inverted pyramid, whereas a distended bladder can have the appearance of an inflated balloon. The bladder neck refers to the inferior portion of the bladder as it approaches the urethra.

Bladder rupture can occur due to blunt or penetrating trauma, and may be intra-peritoneal or extraperitoneal. The anterior and inferior aspects of the bladder are not covered by peritoneum, but the superior and posterior surfaces are.

# Image 6.12

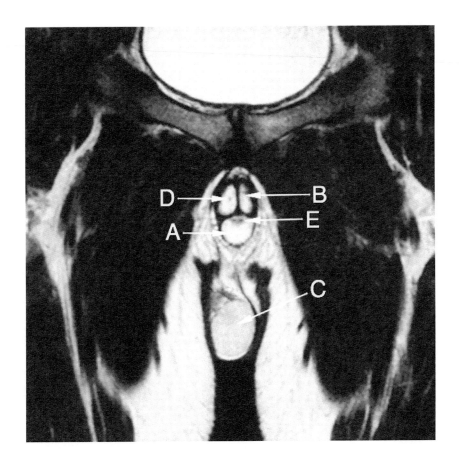

# Image: MR penis (6.12)

## ANSWERS

A   Corpus spongiosum
B   Corpus cavernosum
C   Testis
D   Cavernosal artery
E   Urethra

## LEARNING POINT

In the exam this might be considered a little unfair. In fact the anatomy is relatively simple and easy to learn. The penis is effectively constructed of three tubes surrounded by fascia. The paired dorsal tubes are the corpora cavernosa, which unsurprisingly contain the cavernosal arteries. The central, ventral tube is the corpus spongiosum, which contains the urethra. Each of the corpora is encased separately by the tunica albuginea. Buck's fascia separates the corpora cavernosa from the corpus spongiosum, but incorporates all three within its fascia. The dartos layer contains all three corpora and separates them from the subcutaneous tissues.

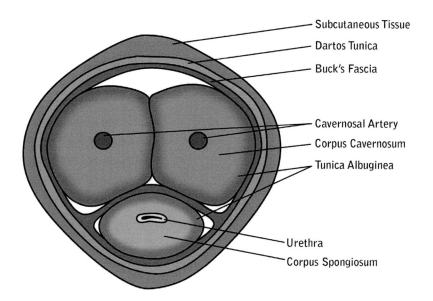

**Figure 6.12a Diagram of penis in cross section.** *Please refer to the colour version in the plate section.*

# Image 6.13

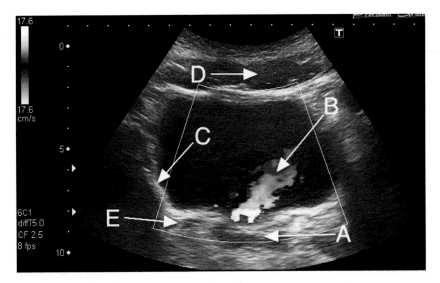

*Please refer to the colour version in the plate section.*

# Image: US transabdominal bladder (6.13)

## ANSWERS

A   Prostate
B   Ureteric jet
C   Bladder wall
D   Rectus abdominis
E   Right ureter

## LEARNING POINT

Ultrasound of the bladder is a common investigation. The ultrasonographic anatomy is no more complex than or different from the earlier examples. This image reminds us of the distal ureteric anatomy.

The ureteric jet is seen to aim superiorly across the bladder. This reminds us that the ureter has travelled inferiorly from the kidney but inserts obliquely through the base of the bladder wall, and is almost facing superiorly at the ureteric orifice. The ureter has the shape of the letter J.

# Image 6.14

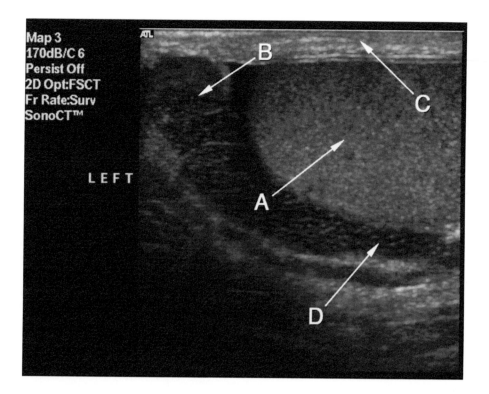

## QUESTIONS

A   Name the structure labelled A.
B   Name the structure labelled B.
C   Name the structure labelled C.
D   Name the structure labelled D.
E   What are the normal testicular dimensions?

# Image: US testis longitudinal (6.14)

## ANSWERS

A   Body of testis
B   Head of epididymis
C   Skin
D   Body of epididymis
E   See below

## LEARNING POINT

Ultrasonic investigation of the testis is a very common examination. It is usually easy to obtain good views of both the testes and the epididymides. The testes are oval shaped and measure approximately 3 cm in length and 2.5 cm in diameter. The seminiferous tubules combine to form the rete testis, and exit the testis at the mediastinum. The mediastinum is an invagination of the tunica albuginea and also serves as the entrance to the testicle for the vessels. The epididymis consists of a head, body and tail. It can be found at the posterior surface of the testicle and is continuous with the vas deferens.

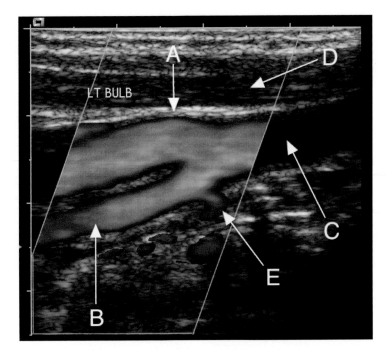

**Image 1.12**

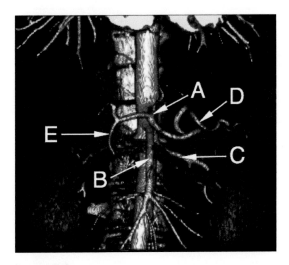

**Image 5.4**

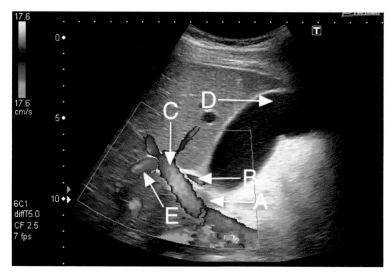

Image 5.12

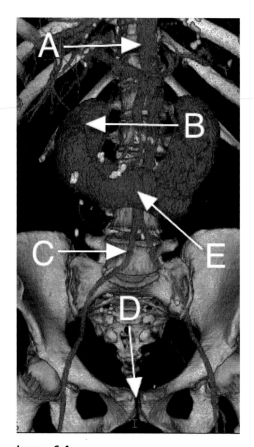

Image 6.4

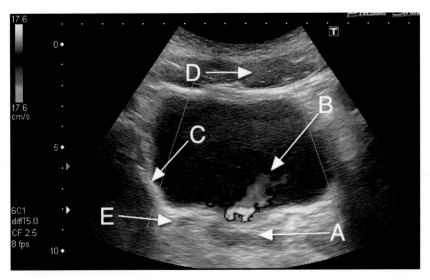

**Image 6.13**

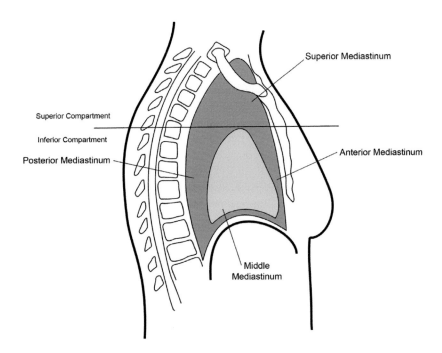

**Figure 2.3a Diagram of mediastinal compartments.**

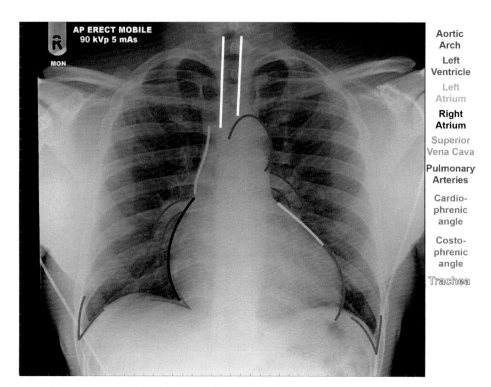

**AP ERECT MOBILE**
90 kVp 5 mAs

MON

Aortic
Arch

Left
Ventricle

Left
Atrium

**Right
Atrium**

Superior
Vena Cava

Pulmonary
Arteries

Cardio-
phrenic
angle

Costo-
phrenic
angle

Trachea

**Figure 2.13a Diagram line drawing of heart borders.**

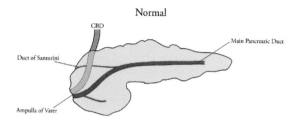

Normal

CBD

Duct of Santorini

Main Pancreatic Duct

Ampulla of Vater

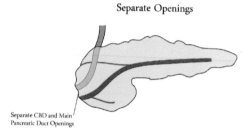

Separate Openings

Separate CBD and Main
Pancreatic Duct Openings

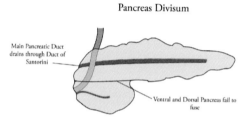

Pancreas Divisum

Main Pancreatic Duct
drains through Duct of
Santorini

Ventral and Dorsal Pancreas fail to
fuse

**Figure 5.2a  Diagram of pancreatic variations.**

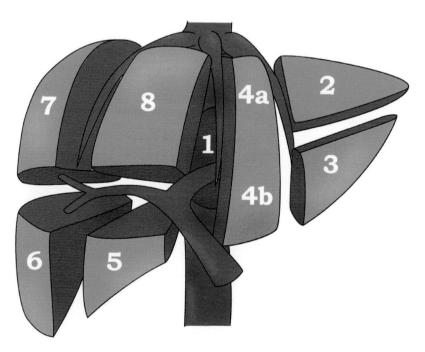

**Figure 5.6a Diagram of liver segments.**

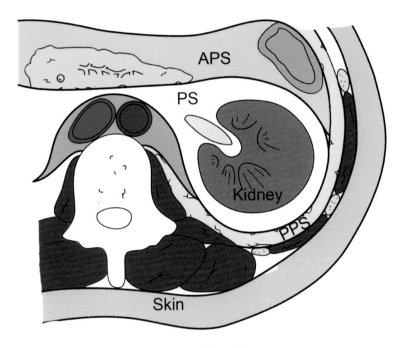

Figure 6.5a Diagram of fascial trifurcation.

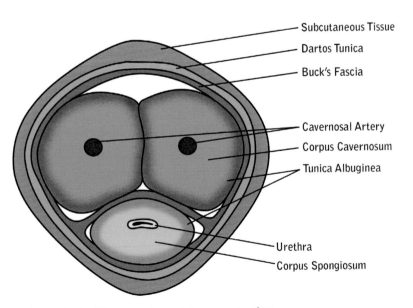

Figure 6.12a Diagram of penis in cross section.

# Chapter 7
# Gynaecological and obstetric

# Image 7.1

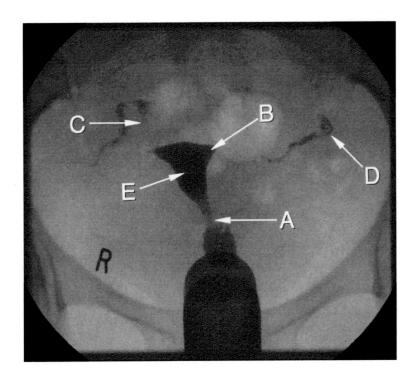

# Image: XR hysterosalpingogram (7.1)

## ANSWERS

A   Cervix
B   Cornu
C   Fallopian tube
D   Ampulla of uterine tube
E   Body of uterus

## LEARNING POINT

Uterine malformation affects around 7% of the population, and approximately 14% of women who suffer recurrent miscarriage. Congenital uterine malformation occurs as a result of abnormal Mullerian duct development. A spectrum of variation exists. There may be a uterine septum, or a bicornuate uterus, uterus didelphys (double uterus), unicornuate uterus (single-sided uterus), or complete uterine agenesis.

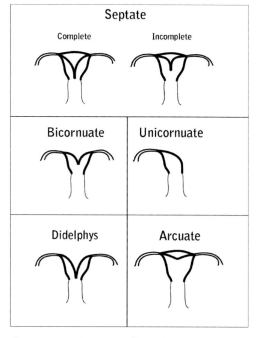

Figure 7.1a Diagram of uterine variants.

# Image 7.2

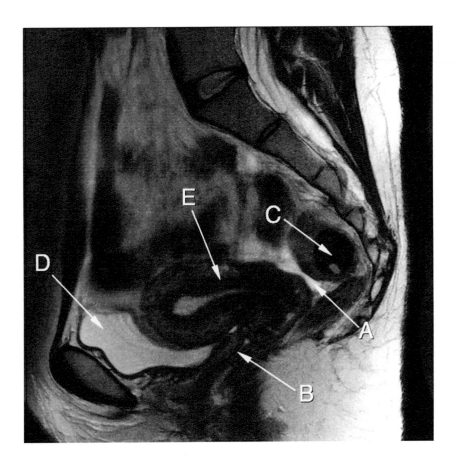

# Image: MR female pelvis sagittal (7.2)

## ANSWERS

A   Pouch of Douglas
B   Vagina
C   Rectum
D   Bladder
E   Uterus

## LEARNING POINT

The pouch of Douglas (or recto-uterine pouch) is an intraperitoneal cavity that lies, as the name suggests, between the rectum and the uterus. It usually represents a potential space, but is often the site of pathology. As the most dependent part of the intraperitoneal cavity, the pouch of Douglas is often the site of pooled blood, ascites or pus.

# Image 7.3

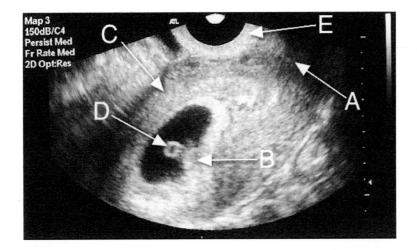

# Image: Transvaginal ultrasound – early pregnancy (7.3)

## ANSWERS

A   Cervix
B   Fetal pole
C   Uterus
D   Yolk sac
E   Vaginal wall

## LEARNING POINT

The gestational sac is used to identify an intrauterine pregnancy prior to the embryo being visualised. The yolk sac is the first visible entity within the gestational sac, and can be seen at about 5 weeks. The bean-shaped fetal pole develops adjacent to the yolk sac and is connected by the vitelline duct to the fetal midgut. The fetal pole becomes the embryo, and by about the ninth gestational week the vitelline duct should obliterate. In approximately 2% of the population the duct fails to close properly and gives rise to a Meckel's diverticulum.

# Image 7.4

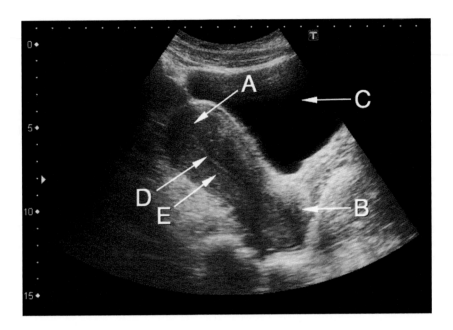

# Image: US female pelvis transabdominal (7.4)

## ANSWERS

A   Uterine fundus.
B   Cervix
C   Bladder
D   Endometrium
E   Myometrium

## LEARNING POINT

The normal position of the uterus is anteverted and anteflexed. The uterus consists mostly of smooth muscle termed the myometrium. Within the centre of the myometrium is the endometrium. The endometrium lines the uterine cavity and varies in thickness throughout the menstrual cycle. In a postmenopausal woman a double-layer thickness of less than 5 mm is regarded as within the normal limits of endometrial thickness.

# Image 7.5

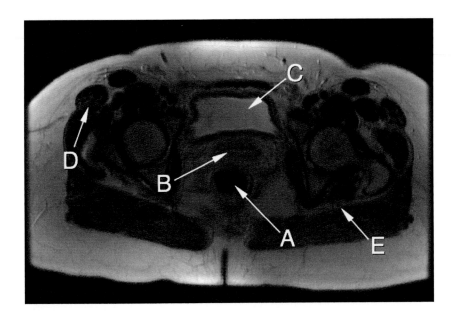

# Image: MR pelvis axial (7.5)

## ANSWERS

A   Rectum
B   Vagina
C   Bladder
D   Right tensor fascia lata
E   Left sciatic nerve

## LEARNING POINT

Assessment of the female pelvis can be subdivided into three functional units. The anterior compartment contains the bladder and urethra, the middle compartment contains the vagina, and the posterior compartment contains the rectum. Each compartment has a fascial and muscular support mechanism. Assessing the competence of these support mechanisms via MR can aid the diagnosis and management of pelvic floor weakness and potential prolapse.

# Image 7.6

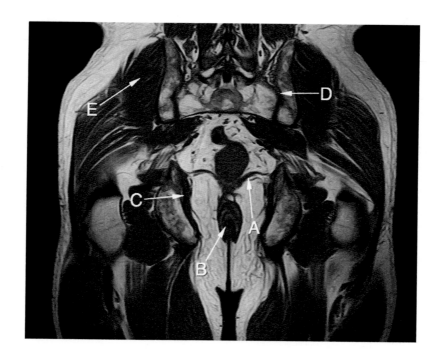

# Image: MR pelvis coronal (7.6)

## ANSWERS

A   Levator ani
B   Anal canal
C   Right obturator internus
D   Left sacroiliac joint
E   Right gluteus maximus

## LEARNING POINT

The levator ani muscle group consists of the paired iliococcygeus and pubococcygeus muscles, together with the U-shaped puborectalis muscle. The levator ani, with the help of the coccygeus, forms the pelvic diaphragm. The pelvic diaphragm provides a sling across the pelvic floor and offers support to the pelvic organs whilst allowing the urethra, vagina and anus to pass through.

The levator ani forms the roof of the ischiorectal fossa, allowing for its demarcation on this coronal image.

# Image 7.7

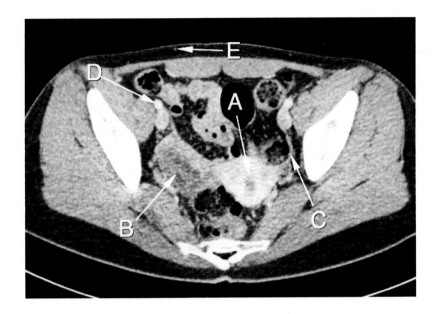

# Image: CT pelvis axial (7.7)

## ANSWERS

A   Uterus
B   Right ovary
C   Left broad ligament
D   Right external iliac artery
E   Left inferior epigastric artery

## LEARNING POINT

Variable position of the ovaries can sometimes make their identification on CT a little tricky. The uterus is normally easy to find, and then the broad ligament should lead you towards the ovary.

The broad ligament is formed by a peritoneal fold that extends from the uterus to the pelvic sidewall. It contains the Fallopian tube, the uterine and ovarian arteries, and the round ligament. The ovary lies adjacent to, but not strictly inside, the broad ligament.

# Chapter 8
# Spine

# Image 8.1

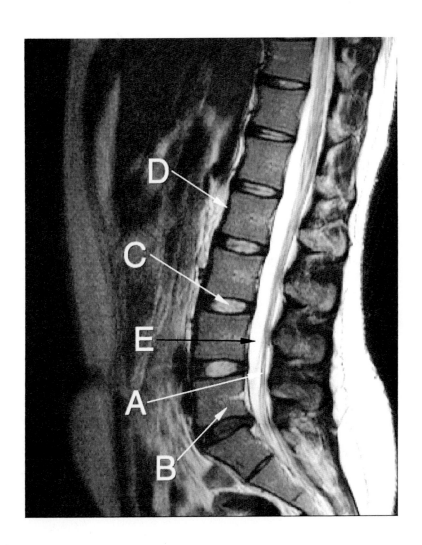

# Image: MR lumbar spine sagittal midline (8.1)

## ANSWERS

A   Cauda equina
B   Vertebral body of L5
C   L3/4 intervertebral disc
D   Anterior longitudinal ligament
E   Caudal lumbar thecal sac

## LEARNING POINT

In adults the spinal cord terminates between T12 and L2, but generally between L1 and L2. The spinal nerves for the lumbar, sacral and coccygeal regions descend from the cord at a higher level as the cauda equina, and exit the central spinal canal inferior to the pedicles of their respective levels (i.e. the L3 spinal nerves will exit beneath the pedicle of L3).

The anterior longitudinal ligament attaches to the anterior aspect of the vertebral bodies and intervertebral discs from the base of the skull, caudally to the anterior surface of the sacrum. Likewise, the posterior longitudinal ligament runs the length of the vertebral canal, attaching to the posterior aspect of the vertebral bodies and intervertebral discs, forming the anterior border of the central vertebral canal itself.

# Image 8.2

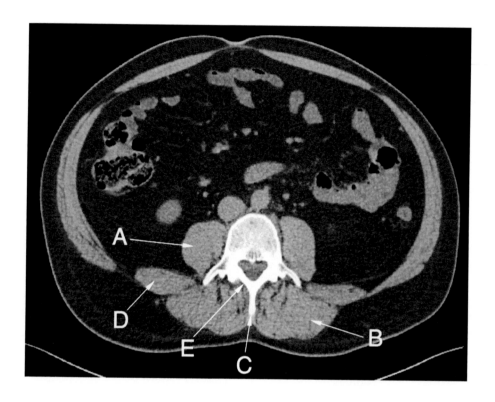

# Image: CT/MR thoraco-lumbar spine axial (8.2)

## ANSWERS

A   Right psoas major
B   Left erector spinae muscles
C   Spinous process
D   Right quadratus lumborum
E   Lamina

## LEARNING POINT

In the thoracolumbar region the erector spinae muscle group consists of three longitudinal bands of muscle running between the angles of the ribs and the spinous processes. From medial to lateral these are called the spinalis, longissimus and iliocostalis. This is rarely relevant clinically, and the term 'erector spinae' will often suffice.

The psoas major muscle arises from the lateral aspects of the vertebral bodies and intervertebral discs of T12–L5, as well as the transverse processes of L1–L5. On axial slice imaging, the left and right psoas muscles appear as ovoid structures running the length of the lateral aspect of the lumbar vertebral bodies.

# Image 8.3

This section has been obtained at the L4/5 intervertebral disc level.

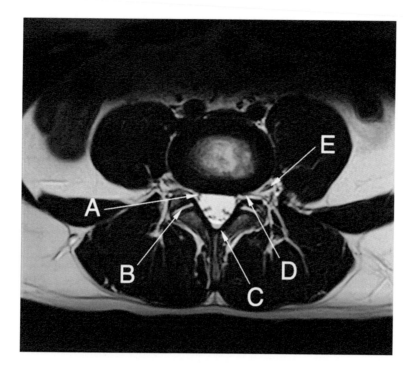

# Image: MR lumbar spine axial (8.3)

## ANSWERS

A   Right traversing L5 nerve root
B   Right L4/5 facet joint
C   Ligamentum flavum
D   Left lateral recess
E   Left L4 exiting spinal nerve

## LEARNING POINT

It is important to grasp lumbar spinal nerve anatomy in order to make any interpretation of which levels are being affected by a particular pathology. Using this case as an example, at the L4/5 intervertebral disc level the exiting nerve roots running out of the exit foramen will be the L4 nerve roots. However, the traversing nerve roots leaving the thecal sac on their way to the lateral recesses (and thence on to their respective exit foramina) are the L5 nerve roots.

These rules hold true for levels below the cervical spine. For example, at the T12/L1 disc level the exiting nerve root is T12, but the L1 nerve root is waiting to leave, making its way centrally from the thecal sac and on to the lateral recesses.

This distinction is important when one is confronted with a disc protrusion, as a central disc will probably affect the traversing roots, whereas a lateral disc will affect the root which is already in or leaving the intervertebral exit foramen.

# Image 8.4

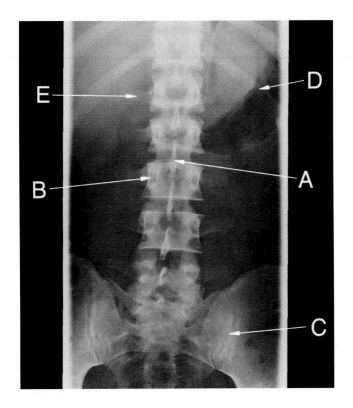

# Image: XR lumbar spine AP (8.4)

## ANSWERS

A   Spinous process of second lumbar vertebra
B   Right pedicle of third lumbar vertebra
C   Left sacro-iliac joint
D   Left 12th rib
E   Right transverse process of first lumbar vertebra

## LEARNING POINT

On an AP projection the pedicles appear bilaterally as ovoid 'eyes' halfway down the height of the vertebral body. They should be sought when reviewing a spinal radiograph, as they are often the site of metastatic deposits.

Be careful to count the number of lumbar vertebrae. Approximately 5% of the population have an anomalous sixth lumbar vertebra.

# Image 8.5

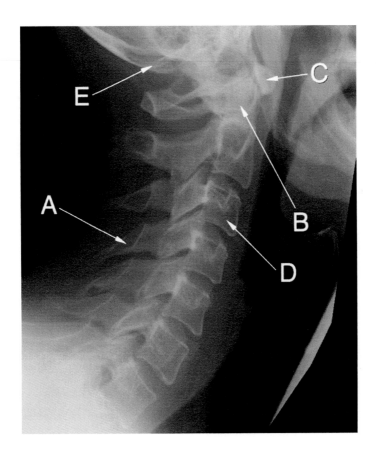

# Image: XR cervical spine lateral (8.5)

## ANSWERS

A   Spinous process of fourth cervical vertebra
B   Dens/odontoid peg
C   Anterior arch of atlas (C1)
D   Vertebral body of third cervical vertebra
E   Occiput/occipital bone

## LEARNING POINT

Four lines should be considered when evaluating a lateral cervical spine radiograph for normal anatomy. These are the anterior and posterior longitudinal lines (along the anterior and posterior borders of the vertebral bodies), and then the spinolaminar line (along the anterior aspect of the spinous process/laminae) and the spinous process line. These lines should be smooth and continuous with no steps.

   In an adult the normal anterior atlanto–dens interval is less than 3 mm. In a child the distance is said to be normal if it is less than 5 mm.

# Image 8.6

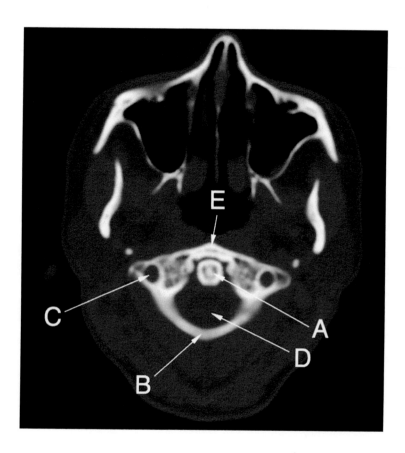

# Image: CT atlanto-axial joint axial (8.6)

## ANSWERS

A   Dens/odontoid peg of axis
B   Posterior arch of atlas (C1)
C   Right foramen transversarium of atlas
D   Vertebral canal/spinal cord
E   Anterior arch of atlas (C1)

## LEARNING POINT

The atlas is a ring-shaped vertebra that lacks a vertebral body. There are two lateral masses connected by anterior and posterior arches. The atlas articulates via superior and inferior facets to the occipital condyles above and the second cervical vertebra below. The anterior arch of the atlas also articulates with the odontoid process of the axis (C2).

The foramina transversaria are small holes found bilaterally in the transverse processes of the cervical vertebrae. These allow the passage of the vertebral artery (and veins) from the thorax to the cranium.

# Image 8.7

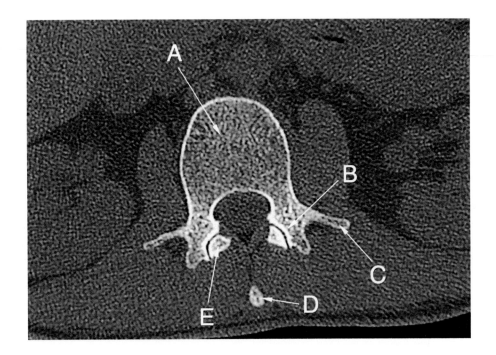

# Image: CT lumbar spine axial (8.7)

## ANSWERS

A  Vertebral body
B  Superior facet
C  Transverse process
D  Spinous process
E  Inferior facet

## LEARNING POINT

Typically each vertebra articulates with another through four synovial facet joints – bilaterally, superiorly and inferiorly. On an axial section through the spine, when one has to decipher the components of the facet joint, the inferior facet will always appear posterior to the facet joint. Conversely, the superior facet is located anteriorly.

# Image 8.8

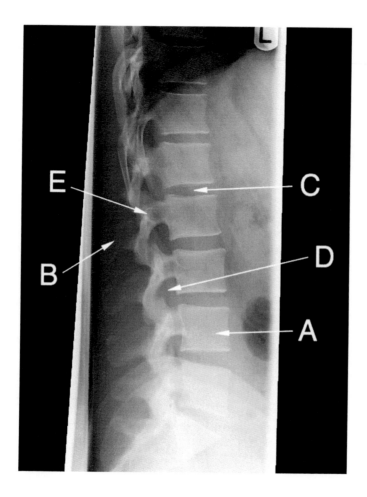

# Image: XR lumbar spine lateral (8.8)

## ANSWERS

A    Vertebral body of fourth lumbar vertebra
B    Spinous process of second lumbar vertebra
C    Intervertebral disc space at L1/2 level
D    Intervertebral foramen at L3/4 level
E    Transverse process of second lumbar vertebra

## LEARNING POINT

Viewing the lumbar vertebral column on a lateral view in the adult should normally show a gentle anterior-facing convexity. This is called the lumbar lordosis. It is a secondary curvature of the spine, which compensates for the primary anterior concavity of the embryological spine, and brings the centre of gravity into a vertical line.

# Image 8.9

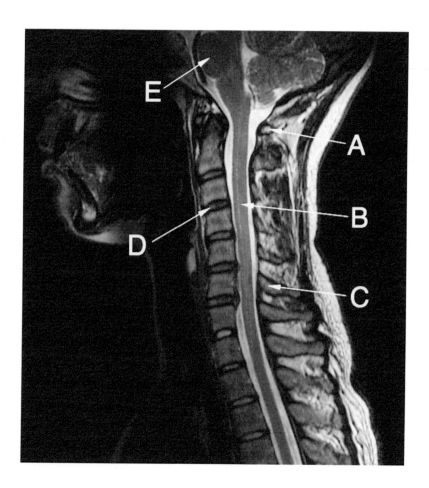

# Image: MR cervical spine sagittal (8.9)

## ANSWERS

A Posterior arch of atlas (C1)
B Cervical spinal cord
C Spinous process of sixth cervical vertebra
D Intervertebral disc of third/fourth cervical vertebrae
E Pons

## LEARNING POINT

Remember that there are eight cervical spinal nerves and only seven cervical vertebrae. The nomenclature of the cervical nerves is therefore slightly different to that of more caudal regions, as the first cervical nerve emerges between the occiput and the atlas (C1). Similarly, the C2 nerves emerge above the second cervical vertebra, and so on. The C8 nerves exit the vertebral canal at the C8/T1 level. Therefore the T1 nerve exits below the first thoracic vertebra and not above it, as in the cervical spine.

# Image 8.10

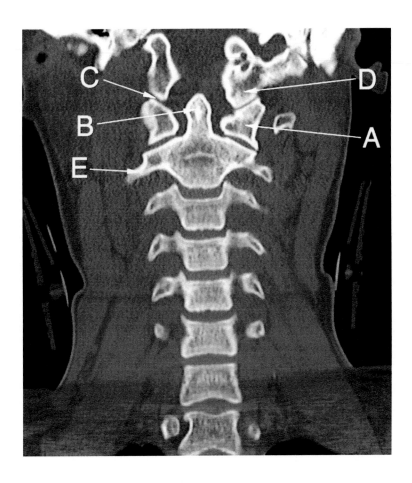

# Image: CT cervical spine sagittal (8.10)

## ANSWERS

A   Left lateral mass of the atlas (C1)
B   Dens/odontoid peg
C   Right atlanto-occipital joint
D   Left occipital condyle
E   Right transverse process of axis (C2)

## LEARNING POINT

The atlanto-occipital joint allows articulation between the atlas and the occipital condyles. It allows forward flexion and extension of the head on the neck, as well as a few degrees of lateral flexion. The atlas and occipital condyles are connected by anterior and posterior atlanto-occipital membranes, two lateral atlanto-occipital ligaments and the atlanto-occipital joint capsule.

# Chapter 9
# Upper limb

## Image 9.1

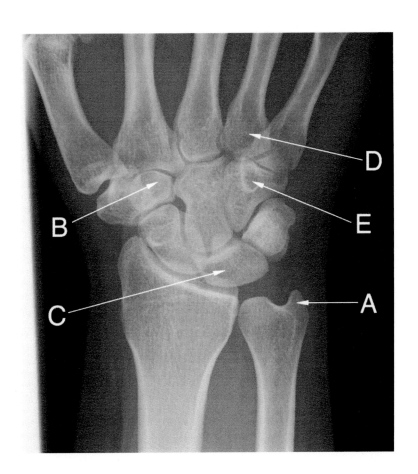

# Image: XR wrist DP (9.1)

## ANSWERS

A   Ulnar styloid
B   Trapezoid
C   Lunate
D   Base of ring finger metacarpal
E   Hook of hamate

## LEARNING POINT

The mnemonic below is quite useful for remembering the bones of the wrist, starting at the scaphoid and moving in the ulnar direction along the proximal row, and then radially along the distal row of carpal bones:

| | |
|---|---|
| Students | Scaphoid |
| Like | Lunate |
| To | Triquetral |
| Party | Pisiform |
| Hangovers | Hamate |
| Cause | Capitate |
| Terrible | Trapezoid |
| Tutorials | Trapezium |

There are much ruder versions, but they are probably unprintable!

# Image 9.2

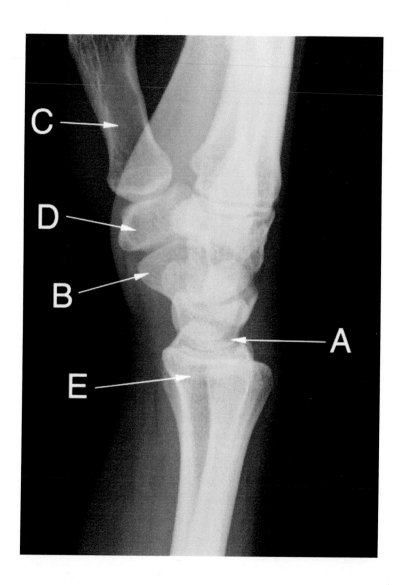

# Image: XR wrist lateral (9.2)

## ANSWERS

A   Lunate
B   Scaphoid
C   Thumb metacarpal
D   Trapezium
E   Distal radius

## LEARNING POINT

The lateral wrist radiograph is an awkward one! There's no real way round this – you just have to get used to looking at them. Knowing the subtle prominences and projections will help.

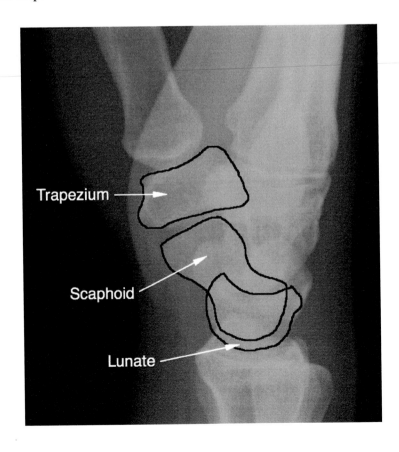

# Image 9.3

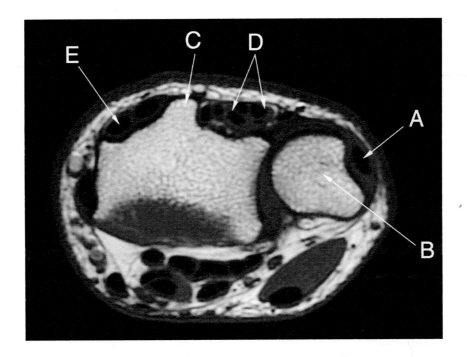

# Image: MR wrist axial (9.3)

## ANSWERS

A   Extensor carpi ulnaris tendon
B   Head of the ulna
C   Lister's tubercle
D   Extensor digitorum tendons
E   Extensor carpi radialis longus tendon

## LEARNING POINT

The wrist MRI is another daunting prospect at first. In terms of the extensor tendons, the best thing to do is to divide the tendons into their anatomical compartments.
    From the radial to the ulnar side, the compartments are as follows:

I       Abductor pollicis longus (APL)
        Extensor pollicis brevis (EPB)

II      Extensor carpi radialis longus (ECRL)
        Extensor carpi radialis brevis (ECRB)

III     Extensor pollicis longus (EPL)
        Remember that moving distally away from Lister's tubercle, the EPL tendon passes over the tendons of compartment II to lie more radially.

IV      Extensor digitorum (ED)
        Extensor indicis (EI)

V       Extensor digiti minimi (EDM)

VI      Extensor carpi ulnaris (ECU)

Note that the first five tendons (compartments I to III) alternate between longus and brevis.

# Image 9.4

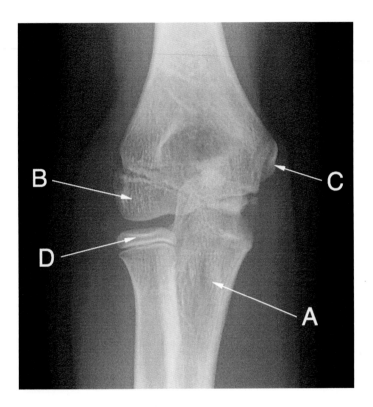

## QUESTIONS

A   Name the structure labelled A.
B   Name the structure labelled B.
C   Name the structure labelled C.
D   Name the structure labelled D.
E   In the paediatric elbow, which is the second ossification centre to appear?

# Image: XR elbow AP paediatric 11-year-old (9.4)

## ANSWERS

A  Ulna
B  Ossification centre for capitellum
C  Ossification centre for medial epicondyle
D  Ossification centre for radial head
E  Radial head

## LEARNING POINT

The sequence in which the ossification centres of the developing elbow appear is very consistent. At birth, the proximal radius and ulna and the distal humerus are entirely cartilaginous. As the child develops, the ossification centres appear in order, at around the same point in time, with girls usually slightly ahead of boys.

A useful and well-known mnemonic is **CRITOL**:

**C**apitellum
**R**adial head
**I**nternal (medial) epicondyle
**T**rochlea
**O**lecranon
**L**ateral epicondyle

# Image 9.5

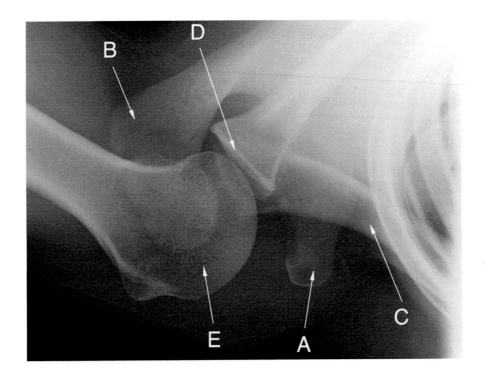

# Image: XR shoulder axial (9.5)

## ANSWERS

A   Coracoid process
B   Acromion
C   Clavicle
D   Glenoid fossa
E   Humeral head

## LEARNING POINT

The axial view of the shoulder is a less commonly performed radiograph. The key is to find the coracoid process and orientate from there. The coracoid is a bony process arising from the scapula, which under normal circumstances points anteriorly (and slightly laterally), and sits just inferior to the lateral part of the clavicle. Therefore on this view one can tell, for example, whether a gleno-humeral dislocation has occurred anteriorly or posteriorly.

# Image 9.6

**QUESTIONS**

A   Name the structure labelled A.
B   Name the structure labelled B.
C   Name the structure labelled C.
D   Name the structure labelled D.
E   Which major muscle tendon attaches at point B?

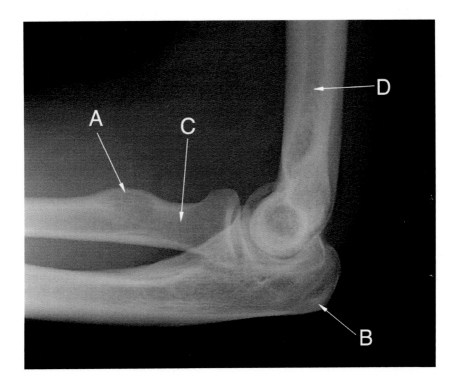

# Image: XR elbow lateral (9.6)

## ANSWERS

A Tuberosity of radius
B Olecranon process of ulna
C Radial neck
D Humerus
E Triceps brachialis

## LEARNING POINT

The lateral elbow view is useful when determining normal joint alignment. If an imaginary line is drawn through the shaft of the radius, and extended through the joint space, the line should pass directly through the capitellum, indicating a congruent radio-capitellar joint. If not, it may indicate a dislocated radial head.

Similarly, a line drawn down the anterior cortex of the humerus should pass through the middle third of the capitellum. If not, this indicates that the capitellum has been displaced posteriorly, and it suggests a possible distal humerus or, in children, a supracondylar fracture.

The tuberosity of the proximal radius is the point of insertion for the biceps brachii tendon. The tuberosity is just on the ulnar side of the proximal radius, and so the action of the biceps is as a flexor of the forearm, but also as a powerful supinator.

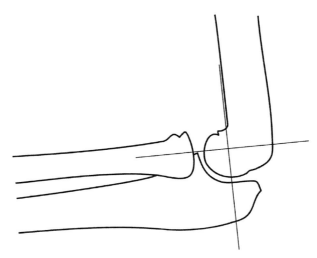

**Figure 9.6a Diagram of radiocapitellar line and anterior humeral line.**

# Image 9.7

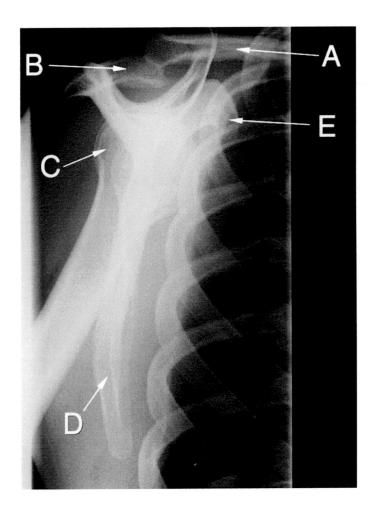

# Image: XR shoulder scapula lateral (9.7)

## ANSWERS

A  Clavicle
B  Acromion
C  Humeral head
D  Blade of scapula
E  Coracoid process

## LEARNING POINT

The scapula lateral view is also known as the 'Y' view, as the confluence of the coracoid and the acromion processes superiorly and the body of the scapula inferiorly forms a Y-shape.

The coracoid is located anteriorly and therefore on this view will be the fork of the Y closest to the chest wall. At the centre of the Y is the glenoid fossa, and therefore the humeral head should be positioned centrally over the Y if correctly located.

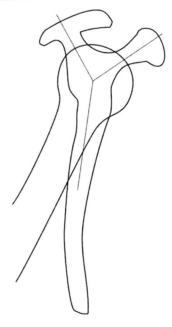

**Figure 9.7a Diagram of scapula y-view.**

# Image 9.8

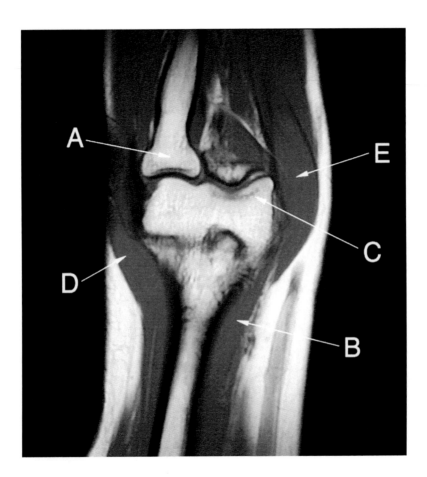

# Image: MR elbow coronal (9.8)

## ANSWERS

A   Radial head
B   Medial head of triceps muscle
C   Trochlea of humerus
D   Brachioradialis
E   Pronator teres

## LEARNING POINT

The triceps brachii, as its name suggests, has three constituent parts. The long head arises from the infraglenoid tubercle. The medial and lateral heads originate from the posterior aspect of the proximal humerus. All three heads converge and insert as a tendon on the olecranon of the ulna.

# Image 9.9

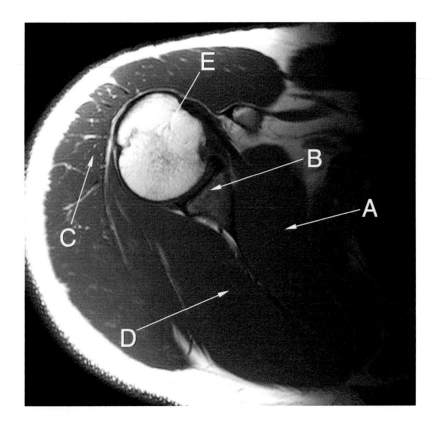

# Image: MR shoulder axial (9.9)

## ANSWERS

A   Subscapularis muscle
B   Glenoid
C   Deltoid muscle
D   Infraspinatus muscle
E   Head of humerus

## LEARNING POINT

The subscapularis arises from the subscapular fossa on the anterior aspect of the scapula. The tendinous portion inserts on the lesser tuberosity of the humerus, and is the only one of the four rotator cuff muscles to do so. The action of the subscapularis is to rotate the arm internally at the gleno-humeral joint.

The infraspinatus muscle originates from the infraspinous fossa (below the spine) on the posterior aspect of the scapula. Another muscle of the rotator cuff group, it attaches on the middle facet of the greater tuberosity, and acts to externally rotate the arm at the shoulder joint.

# Image 9.10

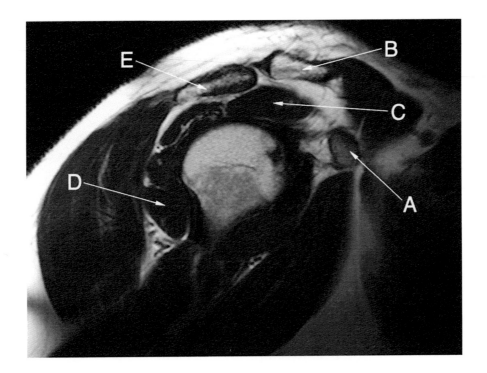

# Image: MR shoulder sagittal oblique (9.10)

## ANSWERS

A   Coracoid process
B   Clavicle
C   Supraspinatus muscle
D   Teres minor muscle
E   Acromion

## LEARNING POINT

The supraspinatus muscle arises from the supraspinous fossa of the posterior aspect of the scapula, passing under the acromion, where the supraspinatus tendon inserts on the superior facet of the greater tuberosity of the humeral head. Due to its high insertion point, the supraspinatus muscle acts to initiate the first 15 degrees of shoulder abduction. After the first few degrees the deltoid muscle becomes the major abductor.

The teres minor muscle, together with the infraspinatus muscle, acts to externally rotate the arm at the gleno-humeral joint. It arises from the lateral part of the lower posterior scapula, and inserts at the inferior facet of the greater tuberosity of the humeral head.

# Image 9.11

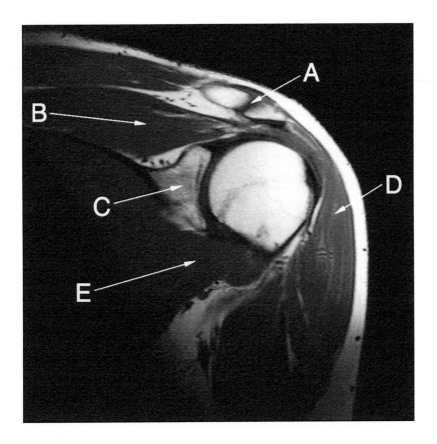

# Image: MR shoulder coronal oblique (9.11)

## ANSWERS

A   Acromioclavicular joint
B   Supraspinatus muscle
C   Glenoid
D   Deltoid muscle
E   Subscapularis muscle

## LEARNING POINT

The deltoid is a large 'delta'-shaped muscle that originates from the anterior aspect of the lateral clavicle, the lateral part of the acromion and the spine of the scapula. It is a superficial muscle that covers the majority of the shoulder joint, and inserts at the deltoid tuberosity (a palpable bony prominence on the lateral aspect of the proximal humeral diaphysis). The action of the deltoid is as an abductor of the arm at the gleno-humeral joint, following initiation by the supraspinatus muscle.

# Image 9.12

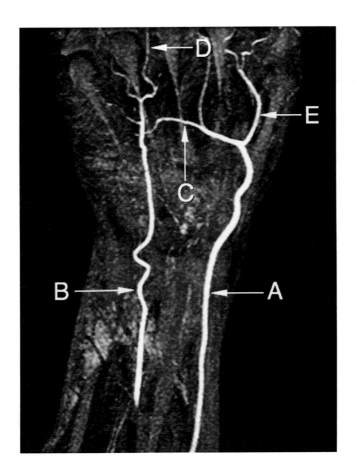

# Image: MR angiogram hand (9.12)

## ANSWERS

A   Radial artery
B   Ulnar artery
C   Palmar arch
D   Digital artery
E   Princeps pollicis artery

## LEARNING POINT

By identifying the metacarpals we can ascertain the orientation of this image. The orientation of the heads of the metacarpals tells us that the thumb must be on the right of the image. Subsequently the radial and ulnar arteries can be accurately recognised and the remaining vessels inferred.

The palmar arch provides an anastomosis between the two major arteries. The princeps pollicis artery supplies the thumb, and the digital arteries supply the fingers.

# Image 9.13

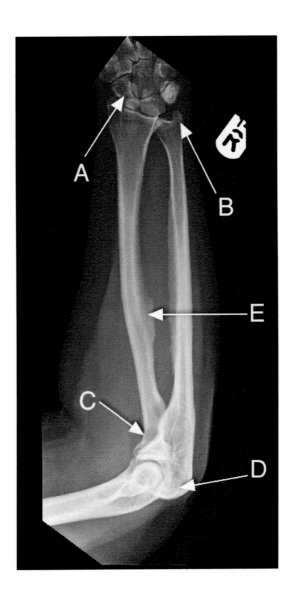

# Image: XR forearm AP (9.13)

## ANSWERS

A   Scaphoid
B   Ulnar styloid
C   Radial head
D   Olecranon
E   Interosseous crest

## LEARNING POINT

The forearm can be regarded as behaving in a similar way to a bony ring structure. The implication of this is that an isolated fracture is rare, as there is usually a second disruption to the ring. Two classical fractures are described, namely the Monteggia fracture and the Galeazzi fracture. Each pattern involves a fracture and a dislocation:

*   Monteggia fracture – ulnar fracture with dislocation of the proximal radius
*   Galeazzi fracture – radial fracture with dislocation of the distal ulna.

The trick is remembering which is which! The following mnemonic is useful:

**M**onteggia **U**lna – **M U** – **M**anchester **U**nited
**G**aleazzi **R**adius – **G R** – **G**lasgow **R**angers

Manchester United play in the **P**remier league, which reminds us that the radial dislocation is **P**roximal.

# Image 9.14

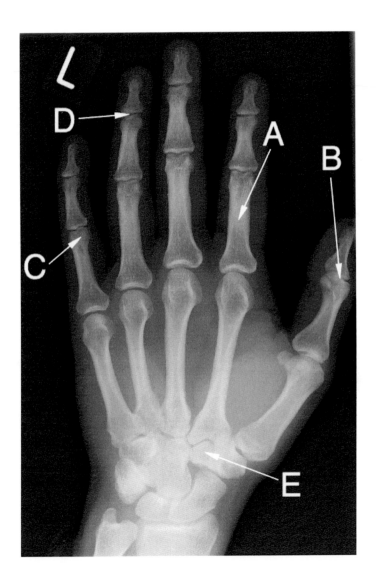

# Image: XR hand DP (9.14)

## ANSWERS

A   Index finger metacarpal
B   Thumb interphalangeal joint
C   Head of proximal phalanx of little finger
D   Distal interphalangeal joint of ring finger
E   Trapezoid

## LEARNING POINT

Common convention dictates that the metacarpals are not numbered, but instead are named according to the digit with which they articulate. Therefore the metacarpal on the most ulnar side is not the fifth metacarpal, but the little finger metacarpal.

Each metacarpal has a base proximally, a shaft, and a head distally. The same is true for the phalanges of each digit. The head of the metacarpal therefore articulates with the base of the proximal phalanx of the digit.

# Image 9.15

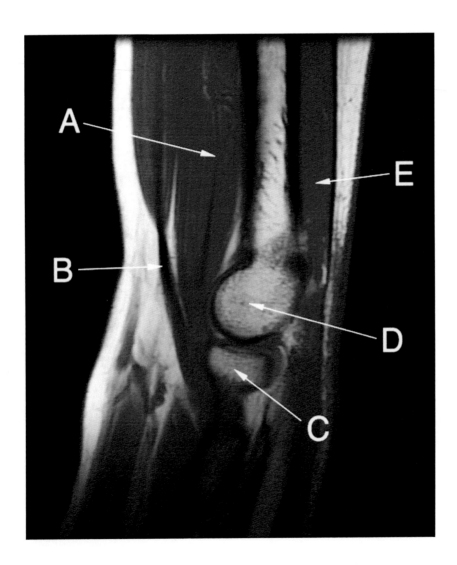

# Image: MR elbow coronal (9.15)

## ANSWERS

A   Brachialis
B   Distal tendon of biceps brachii
C   Radial head
D   Capitellum
E   Lateral head of triceps brachii

## LEARNING POINT

The two heads of the biceps muscle have separate origins. The long head arises from the supraglenoid tubercle as a tendon, and becomes an intra-articular structure passing through the gleno-humeral joint. The short head arises from the coracoid process of the scapula. The two converge to form the two muscle bellies of the biceps brachii. The muscle lies superficial to the coracobrachialis and brachialis in the anterior compartment of the arm. The distal tendon of the biceps inserts at the radial tuberosity.

   Remember that the **B**asilic vein and **B**rachial artery both lie medially at the elbow, with the basilic vein situated more medially and superficially. The cephalic vein lies on the lateral side of the elbow. The two large superficial veins of the upper limb communicate at the elbow via the median cubital vein.

# Image 9.16

## QUESTIONS

A   Name the structure labelled A.
B   Name the structure labelled B.
C   Name the structure labelled C.
D   Name the structure labelled D.
E   What is the name of this region, and which tendons run through it?

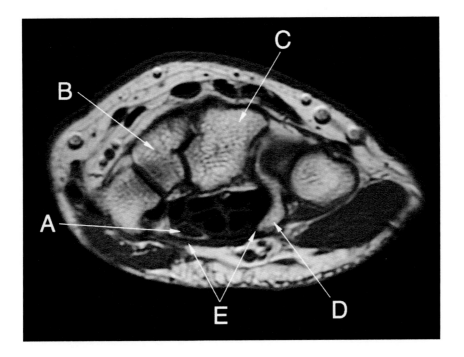

# Image: MR wrist carpal tunnel axial (9.16)

## ANSWERS

A  Median nerve
B  Trapezoid
C  Capitate
D  Hook of hamate
E  Carpal tunnel: flexor digitorum profundus (x 4); flexor digitorum superficialis (x 4); flexor pollicis longus

## LEARNING POINT

The carpal tunnel is a conduit located on the volar aspect of the wrist, which allows the passage of several tendinous structures as well as an important nerve. The posterior and lateral walls are formed by the semicircle created by the two rows of carpal bones. The bases of the arch are formed radially by the tubercles of the trapezium and scaphoid, whilst the hook of the hamate and the pisiform form the ulnar aspect of the arch base. The volar aspect of the tunnel is formed by the thick flexor retinaculum.

In addition to the tendons mentioned above, the median nerve passes through the tunnel on its passage to the hand. This is a common site of entrapment for the nerve, which can lead to carpal tunnel syndrome.

# Chapter 10
# Lower limb

## Image 10.1

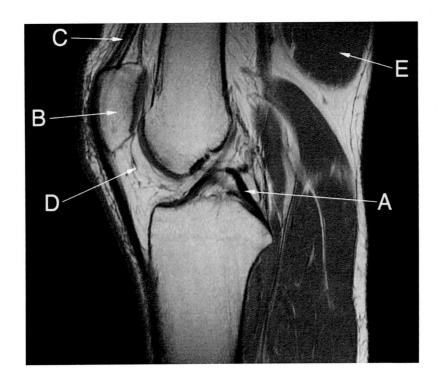

# Image: MRI knee sagittal midline (10.1)

## ANSWERS

A  Posterior cruciate ligament
B  Patella
C  Quadriceps tendon
D  Hoffa's pad/infrapatellar fat pad
E  Semimembranosus

## LEARNING POINT

The cruciate ligaments connect the tibia to the femur. They are called cruciate (cross-shaped) because they cross over each other as they pass from the tibia to the femur.

The anterior cruciate ligament passes from the anterior aspect of the intercondylar area of the tibia, posteriorly to the lateral aspect of the intercondylar fossa. Conversely, the posterior cruciate ligament passes from the posterior part of the intercondylar eminence anteriorly to the medial aspect of the intercondylar fossa of the femur.

On an MRI scan of the knee, the anterior cruciate ligament appears as a fibrillated structure, whereas the posterior cruciate ligament has a more solid, simple architecture.

# Image 10.2

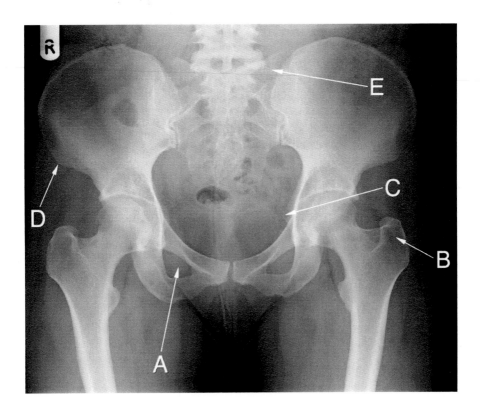

# Image: XR pelvis AP (10.2)

## ANSWERS

A   Right obturator foramen
B   Left greater trochanter
C   Left ischial spine
D   Right anterior inferior iliac spine
E   Left superior ala of sacrum

## LEARNING POINT

The obturator foramen, which is mostly closed by a membrane in life, provides a route of transmission between the pelvis and the medial aspect of the thigh. The obturator nerve and the obturator artery and vein pass through this foramen.

    The anterior inferior iliac spine is the point of origin for the straight head of the rectus femoris muscle. The reflected head of rectus femoris arises from the ilium just superior to the acetabulum. Together with the vastus muscles, these form the most superficial of the quadriceps muscle group.

# Image 10.3

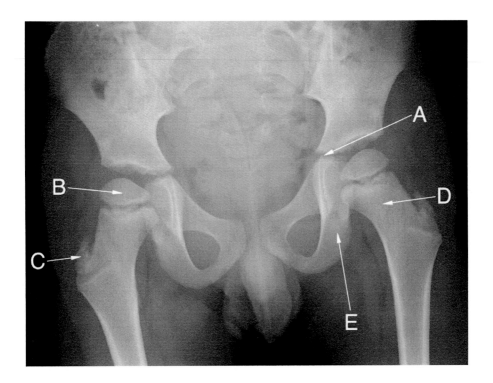

# Image: XR pelvis AP paediatric 5-year-old (10.3)

## ANSWERS

A   Left triradiate cartilage
B   Right capital femoral epiphysis
C   Right ossification centre for greater trochanter
D   Left neck of femur
E   Left ischium

## LEARNING POINT

The triradiate cartilage is a Y-shaped structure that connects the three bones that make up the bony acetabulum in childhood, namely the pubis, ischium and ilium. Fusion of these bones begins to take place at about 16 years of age.

The centre for the head of the femur (or capital femoral epiphysis) normally appears at about 4 to 6 months of age. It fuses between the ages of 14 and 18 years. These ages are important to bear in mind when considering pathology in the paediatric hip, such as developmental dysplasia of the hip (DDH) and slipped capital femoral epiphysis.

# Image 10.4

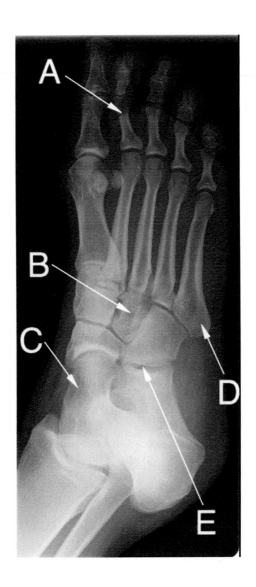

# Image: XR foot DP oblique (10.4)

## ANSWERS

A   Proximal phalanx of second toe
B   Lateral cuneiform
C   Talus
D   Base/styloid of fifth metatarsal
E   Calcaneo-cuboid joint

## LEARNING POINT

It is easier to remember the names of the bones in the foot if you look at the shape of them. The cuboid is obviously cube-shaped, the navicular bone (navy) resembles a boat in shape, and the cuneiforms (medial/intermediate/lateral) derive their name from the Latin for 'wedge.'

The intertarsal joints allow movement between the tarsal bones. The synovial joints of most clinical relevance are the calcaneo-cuboid joint, the talocalcaneo-navicular joint and the subtalar joint (inferior talus–superior calcaneus).

# Image 10.5

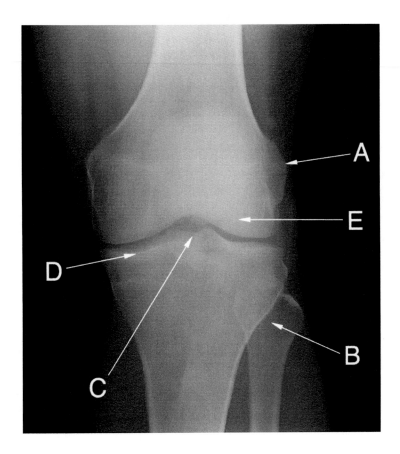

# Image: XR knee AP (10.5)

## ANSWERS

A   Lateral epicondyle of femur
B   Head of fibula
C   Tubercles of intercondylar eminence
D   Medial condyle of tibia/medial tibial plateau
E   Lateral femoral condyle

## LEARNING POINT

The epicondyles of the femur are non-articulating prominences formed for the attachment of the collateral ligaments.

The medial and lateral femoral condyles articulate with the respective condyles of the tibia. The outer margins of the tibial condyles relate to the menisci of the knee joint.

# Image 10.6

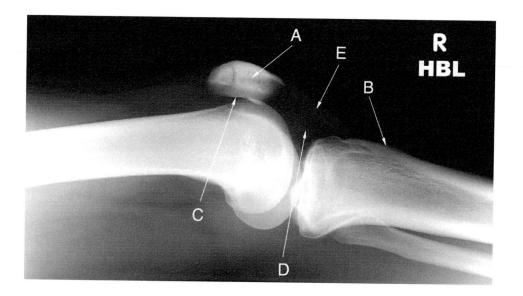

# Image: XR knee lateral (10.6)

## ANSWERS

A   Patella
B   Tibial tuberosity
C   Retropatellar articular surface
D   Hoffa's fat pad
E   Patellar tendon

## LEARNING POINT

A bipartite/multipartite patella is a relatively common congenital anomaly, found in approximately 1% of the population. Essentially the patella has a congenital fragmentation or synchondrosis, failing to fuse, and leading to a patella with two or sometimes more fragments. It is important to know of the existence of bipartite/multipartite patellas, as they can be mistaken for fractures in the acute setting, and can also cause symptoms themselves.

The tibial tuberosity is the bony prominence on the anterior aspect of the proximal tibia that forms the insertion point for the patellar tendon. The patellar tendon is a continuation of the quadriceps tendon after it has passed distally to the sesamoid patellar bone.

# Image 10.7

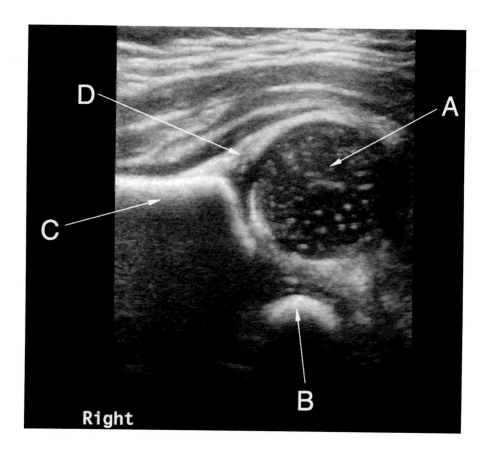

## QUESTIONS

A   Name the structure labelled A.
B   Name the structure labelled B.
C   Name the structure labelled C.
D   Name the structure labelled D.
E   In which plane is this standard image taken?

# Image: US hip longitudinal paediatric (10.7)

## ANSWERS

A   Femoral head (cartilaginous)
B   Ischium
C   Ilium
D   Acetabular roof
E   Coronal

## LEARNING POINT

The femoral head is unossified in infancy, so ultrasound can be used with good effect to visualise it. The femoral head lies within the bony acetabulum. In the imaging plane seen in the figure, the ilium is identified as a straight line superior to the femoral head and parallel to the transducer. Normally, an imaginary line projected from the ilium should bisect the cartilaginous femoral head. The labrum is seen as a hypoechoic rim of tissue between the bony acetabulum and the femoral head.

# Image 10.8

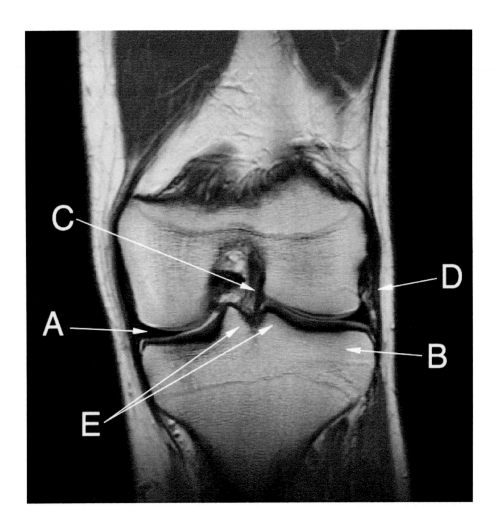

# Image: MRI knee coronal midline (10.8)

## ANSWERS

A   Medial meniscus
B   Lateral tibial plateau/condyle
C   Anterior cruciate ligament
D   Lateral collateral ligament
E   Tubercles of intercondylar eminence

## LEARNING POINT

The menisci are fibrocartilaginous structures that aid the articulation of the femur with the tibia. When viewed in the axial plane, the medial meniscus is 'C'-shaped, whereas the lateral meniscus is more 'O'-shaped. The medial meniscus attaches to the medial collateral ligament, and therefore an injury to one should require close inspection of the other.

The collateral ligaments provide stability to the knee joint. The lateral collateral ligament attaches at the lateral femoral epicondyle, and inferiorly on the lateral surface of the fibular head. Likewise, the medial collateral ligament arises at the medial femoral epicondyle and attaches at the medial margin of the tibia, just posterior to the insertions of the semitendinosus, gracilis and sartorius tendons – the so-called pes anserinus (or goosefoot).

# Image 10.9

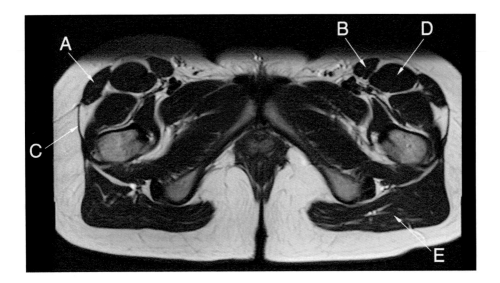

# Image: CT/MRI proximal thigh axial (10.9)

## ANSWERS

A   Right tensor fasciae latae
B   Left sartorius
C   Right iliotibial tract
D   Left rectus femoris
E   Left gluteus maximus

## LEARNING POINT

The sartorius muscle is a long thin muscle that arises from the anterior superior iliac spine and inserts at the pes anserinus (with the gracilis and semitendinosus tendons), located at the antero-medial surface of the proximal tibia. Therefore the muscle belly crosses from lateral to medial on axial imaging, scanning distally down the lower limb.

The function of the sartorius is to flex at the hip and knee joints. The word 'sartorius' is derived from a Latin word meaning 'to tailor', as apparently tailors adopt a cross-legged position when in their sewing posture for their tailoring duties!

The iliotibial tract is a thickening of the deep fascia of the thigh, called the fascia lata (derived from the Latin for 'broad' or 'thick'). The iliotibial tract runs from the tubercle of the iliac crest, and inserts at the lateral aspect of the proximal tibia. Two muscles insert into the iliotibial tract, namely the tensor fasciae latae anteriorly, and the gluteus maximus posteriorly. In combination their purpose is to help to stabilise the knee and hip joints in extension.

# Image 10.10

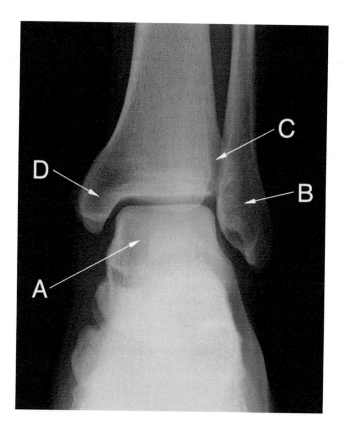

## QUESTIONS

A   Name the structure labelled A.
B   Name the structure labelled B.
C   Name the structure labelled C.
D   Name the structure labelled D.
E   What is the normal distance between the medial surface of the talus and the articular surface of the medial malleolus (medial clear space) on an AP view?

# Image: XR ankle AP (10.10)

## ANSWERS

A   Talus
B   Lateral malleolus (of fibula)
C   Inferior tibio-fibular syndesmosis/joint
D   Medial malleolus
E   4 millimetres or less

## LEARNING POINT

The inferior tibio-fibular syndesmosis is a fibrous joint that prevents the distal tibia and fibula from separating when weight bearing. It is supported by a number of ligaments, which if strained or torn can result in widening of the syndesmosis. The normal distance is 5 millimetres or less. If the distance is any greater than this, diastasis has occurred.

The ankle mortise refers to the structure formed by the tibial plafond and the lateral and medial malleoli. The dome of the talus articulates with these to form the ankle joint. The distance between the medial talus and the articular aspect of the medial malleolus should be 4 mm or less, and should be equal to or less than the distance of the superior tibio-talar clear space.

# Image 10.11

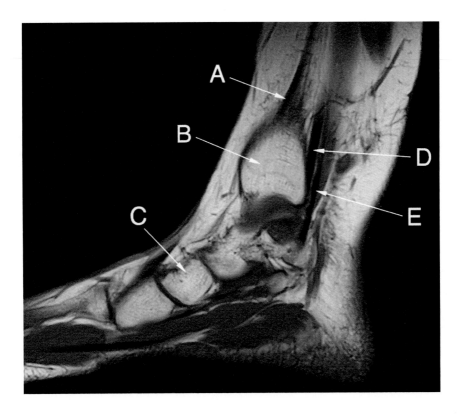

# Image: MR ankle sagittal (medial) (10.11)

## ANSWERS

A    Tibialis anterior tendon
B    Distal tibia
C    Navicular
D    Tibialis posterior tendon
E    Flexor digitorum longus tendon

## LEARNING POINT

There are many tendons and vessels that traverse the ankle joint to reach the foot. Posterior to the medial malleolus deep to the flexor retinaculum lies the tarsal tunnel. Three tendons, two vessels and one nerve run through this tunnel.

Running from the immediate posterior aspect of the medial malleolus, in a posterolateral direction, are the following:

| | |
|---|---|
| **T**om | **T**ibialis posterior tendon |
| **D**ick | Flexor **D**igitorum longus tendon |
| **A**nd | Posterior tibial **A**rtery and accompanying veins, then tibial nerve |
| **Harry** | Flexor **H**allucis longus tendon |

# Image 10.12

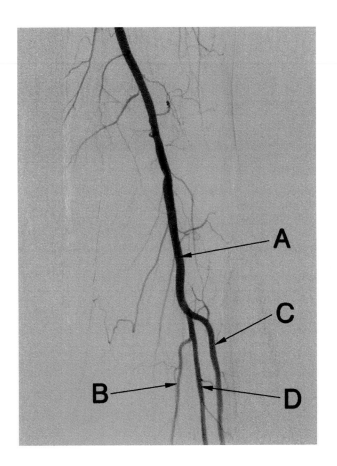

## QUESTIONS

A   Name the structure labelled A.
B   Name the structure labelled B.
C   Name the structure labelled C.
D   Name the structure labelled D.
E   What is the name of the artery that is the continuation of the anterior tibial artery in the foot?

# Image: DSA lower limb AP (10.12)

## ANSWERS

A   Popliteal artery
B   Posterior tibial artery
C   Anterior tibial artery
D   Peroneal artery
E   Dorsalis pedis artery

## LEARNING POINT

The popliteal artery divides into two major branches as it passes deep to the two heads of soleus. These are the anterior tibial artery and the posterior tibial artery. The anterior tibial artery almost immediately passes into and supplies the anterior compartment of the leg.

The posterior tibial artery runs in the deep region of the posterior compartment lying on the muscle bellies of the tibialis posterior and flexor digitorum longus. It eventually passes through the tarsal tunnel, posterior to the medial malleolus.

The peroneal artery branches from the proximal posterior tibial artery, and contrary to its name and common sense, runs in the lateral aspect of the posterior aspect of the posterior compartment adjacent to the fibula. It does, however, give off multiple branches which perforate the intermuscular septum to supply the peroneal muscles.

Looking at an AP projection of the arterial branches of the knee and leg, running from medial to lateral:

Posterior tibial artery → Peroneal artery → Anterior tibial artery

# Image 10.13

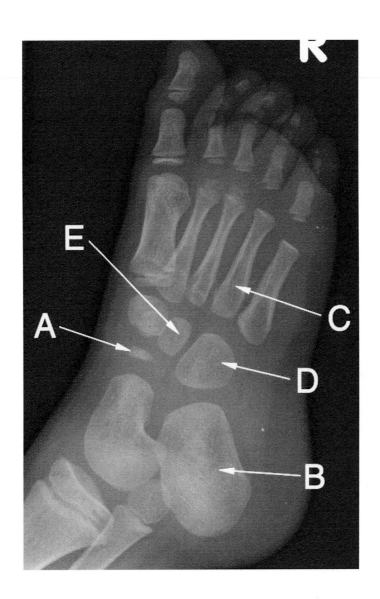

# Image: XR foot DP oblique paediatric 3-year-old (10.13)

## ANSWERS

A   Navicular
B   Calcaneus
C   Fourth metatarsal
D   Cuboid
E   Lateral cuneiform

## LEARNING POINT

Knowing in which order the ossification centres appear in musculoskeletal paediatric radiology is the key to learning the radiographic anatomy.

The ossification centres of the calcaneus, talus and cuboid all appear *in utero*. The lateral cuneiform is the first tarsal bone to ossify postnatally, at 6 months to 1 year. The medial and intermediate cuneiforms ossify much later, at 3 to 4 years of age. The navicular ossification centre also appears at about 3 years.

# Image 10.14

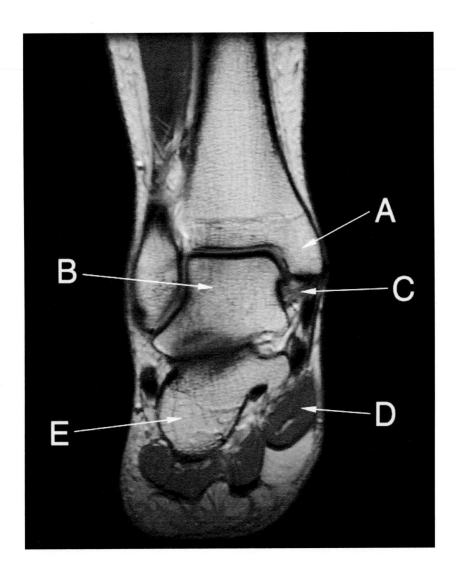

# Image: MR ankle coronal (10.14)

## ANSWERS

A   Medial malleolus
B   Talus
C   Deltoid ligament
D   Abductor hallucis
E   Calcaneus

## LEARNING POINT

The deltoid ligament is a complex structure consisting of four different ligaments which attach the medial aspect of the distal tibia to the medial aspect of the talus and mid- and hindfoot. They are separately named the tibiocalcaneal ligament, the tibionavicular ligament, and the anterior and posterior tibiotalar ligaments.

# Image 10.15

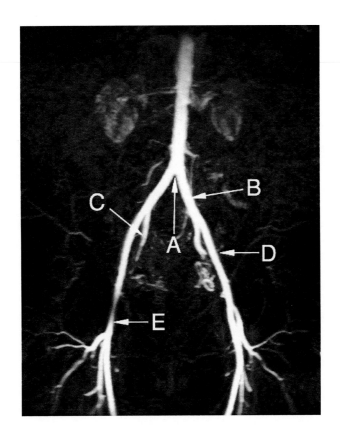

# Image: MRA pelvis (10.15)

## ANSWERS

A   Aortic bifurcation
B   Left common iliac artery
C   Right internal iliac artery
D   Left external iliac artery
E   Right common femoral artery

## LEARNING POINT

The aorta bifurcates at the level of the fourth lumbar vertebra. This bifurcation gives rise to the common iliac arteries. These divide into internal and external iliac arteries at the pelvic brim anterior to the sacroiliac joints. The internal branch courses posteriorly to supply the pelvic contents. The external iliac artery continues to travel inferiorly to supply blood to the leg. As the external iliac artery passes posterior to the inguinal ligament its name changes and it becomes the femoral artery.

It is worth remembering that as the femoral nerve and vessels pass into the femoral canal they have a standard configuration.

From lateral to medial:
Nerve → Artery → Vein

# Image 10.16

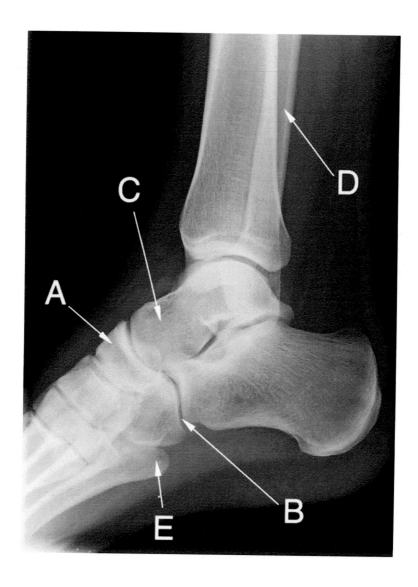

# Image: XR ankle lateral (10.16)

## ANSWERS

A  Navicular
B  Calcaneo-cuboid joint
C  Head of talus
D  Fibula
E  Base/styloid of fifth metatarsal

## LEARNING POINT

The base of the fifth metatarsal is an important bony landmark to appreciate on any radiographs of the foot or ankle. The peroneus brevis muscle, which arises from the lateral surface of the lower part of the fibula, becomes tendinous and passes along the lateral aspect of the calcaneus to insert at the lateral part of the base of the fifth metatarsal. Its normal function is to evert the foot. An inversion injury can cause an avulsion fracture of the fifth metatarsal styloid at the attachment of the peroneus brevis.

# Image 10.17

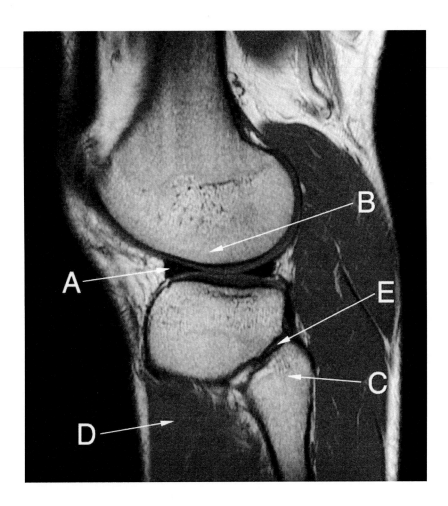

# Image: MRI knee parasagittal lateral (10.17)

## ANSWERS

A   Anterior horn of lateral meniscus
B   Lateral femoral condyle
C   Head of fibula
D   Tibialis anterior
E   Proximal tibiofibular joint

## LEARNING POINT

In a parasagittal plane the menisci have a 'bow-tie'-shaped appearance, with an anterior and posterior horn easily visible between the articulating surfaces of the tibial and femoral condyles.

The tibialis anterior muscle is a strong dorsiflexor of the foot. Its large muscle belly lies within the anterior compartment of the leg, originating proximally from the lateral surface of the triangular-shaped tibia. It is the most medial and anterior of the muscles in this compartment.

# Image 10.18

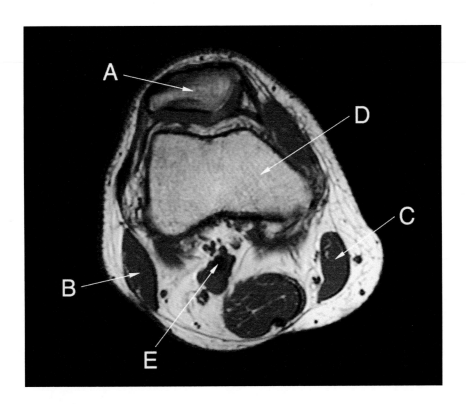

# Image: MRI knee axial (10.18)

## ANSWERS

A   Patella
B   Biceps femoris
C   Sartorius
D   Femur
E   Popliteal artery

## LEARNING POINT

The patella is a sesamoid bone – one which lies within a tendon. In this instance the tendon is the quadriceps tendon as it passes from the thigh to the leg. Once distal to the patella, the tendon is then named the patellar tendon or ligament.

The posterior surface of the patella articulates with the anterior surface of the femoral condyles. The patella is asymmetrical in the axial view. The posterior patellar surface consists of a shorter more vertical medial facet, and a longer more horizontal lateral facet. As a result, the posterior articulating surface resembles a 'tick' shape, or a reverse tick if one is considering the right patellofemoral joint. It is important to remember this, as it should help you to work out which is the medial side and which is the lateral side of an axial view of the knee at this level.

# Image 10.19

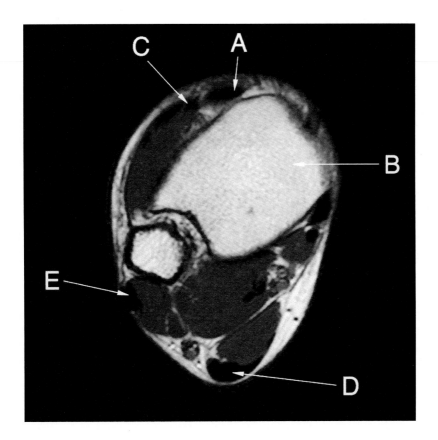

# Image: MR ankle axial (10.19)

## ANSWERS

A   Tibialis anterior tendon
B   Tibia
C   Extensor hallucis tendon
D   Achilles tendon/tendo calcaneus
E   Tibialis posterior tendon

## LEARNING POINT

The tendons of three of the muscles within the anterior compartment of the leg cross the ankle joint lying antero-laterally to the tibia. From medial to lateral they are the tibialis anterior, the extensor hallucis longus and the extensor digitorum longus. The tibialis anterior is a strong dorsiflexor of the foot, inserting on the medial cuneiform and the base of the first metatarsal. The extensor hallucis longus and extensor digitorum longus insert into the distal, and in the case of the extensor digitorum longus, the middle phalanges. Their action is to extend the toes.

# Image 10.20

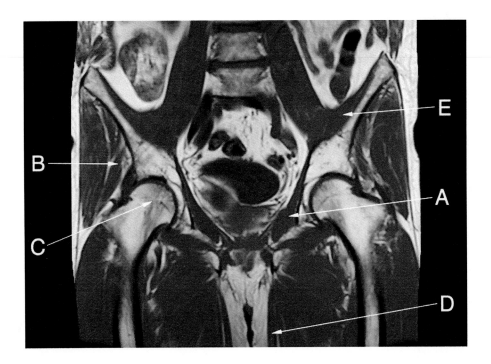

# Image: MR hips coronal (10.20)

## ANSWERS

A   Left obturator internus
B   Right gluteus minimus
C   Right head of femur
D   Left gracilis
E   Left iliacus

## LEARNING POINT

The gracilis muscle is the most medial and superficial muscle within the medial compartment of the thigh. The other muscles in this group are the adductors (brevis, longus and magnus), the pectineus and the obturator externus. The majority of these muscles adduct the hip. The gracilis muscle is recognisable as a thin strap-like muscle that arises from the inferior pubic ramus medially, and descends the length of the thigh to insert on the medial aspect of the proximal tibia (the pes anserinus).

# Image 10.21

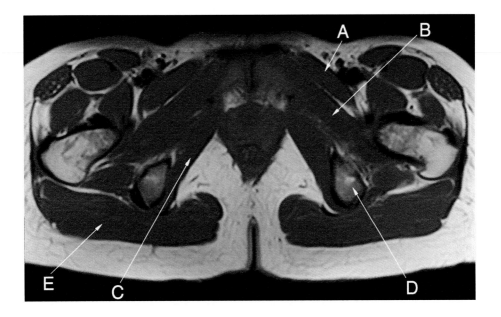

# Image: MR hips axial (10.21)

## ANSWERS

A  Left pectineus
B  Left obturator externus
C  Right obturator internus
D  Left ischial tuberosity
E  Right gluteus maximus

## LEARNING POINT

The pectineus is a flat rectangular muscle that is located anteriorly within the medial compartment of the thigh. On an axial section through the pubic symphysis, the medial origin of the muscle appears at the pectineal line adjacent to the pubic symphysis. It travels laterally and inferiorly, and slightly posterior to the femoral vessels, to attach on a longitudinal line from the lesser trochanter to the linea aspera. Its action is therefore to adduct the hip. There is also a weak flexor component.

# Image 10.22

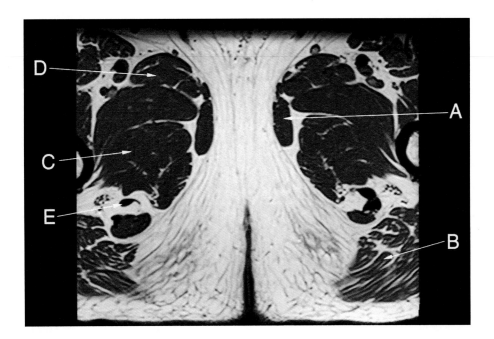

# Image: MR thigh axial (10.22)

## ANSWERS

A   Left gracilis
B   Left gluteus maximus
C   Right adductor magnus
D   Right adductor longus
E   Right sciatic nerve

## LEARNING POINT

There are three named adductor muscles in the medial compartment of the thigh, namely the longus, brevis and magnus. On an axial section through the proximal thigh, the muscle bellies sit in a consistent order from anterior to posterior: longus → brevis → magnus (or **L**ong **B**efore **M**agnus if that's easier to remember).

The adductor magnus muscle consists of a hamstring component and an adductor component. The adductor component arises from the inferior pubic ramus and has a long attachment down the postero-medial aspect of the femur to the medial supra-condylar region. The hamstring component of the adductor magnus arises from the ischial tuberosity and inserts on the adductor tubercle of the medial condyle of the femur. The small gap between the attachments of the two components is termed the adductor hiatus. This is the conduit through which the femoral vessels in the anterior thigh pass posteriorly to continue as the popliteal vessels behind the knee joint.

# Image 10.23

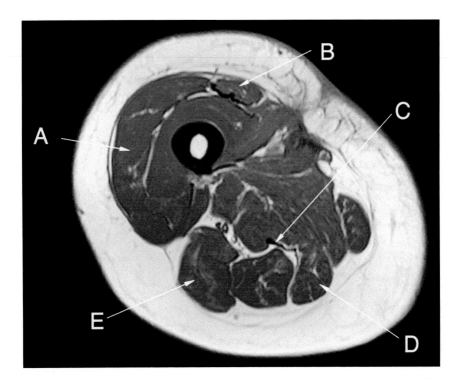

# Image: MR mid-thigh axial (10.23)

## ANSWERS

A  Vastus lateralis
B  Rectus femoris
C  Sciatic nerve
D  Semimembranosus
E  Biceps femoris

## LEARNING POINT

The hamstrings are situated in the posterior compartment of the thigh. The most lateral muscle of the group is the biceps femoris, which consists of a long and short head. The long head arises from the infero-medial aspect of the ischial tuberosity. The origin of the short head is the linea aspera of the femur. The two converge laterally and insert on the head of the fibula. Its major action is to flex the knee joint.

The most medial muscle of the hamstring group at this level is the semimembranosus. It arises from the supero-lateral aspect of the ischial tuberosity, and then descends the thigh, for the most part running deep to the semitendinosus, eventually inserting on the medial and posterior aspect of the medial tibial condyle.

The last muscle of the posterior compartment of the thigh is the semitendinosus, which arises close to the long head of the biceps femoris on the ischial tuberosity. It lies superficial and slightly lateral to the semimembranosus, and just medial to the biceps femoris. It inserts on the medial aspect of the proximal tibia. Together with the semimembranosus it acts to flex the knee joint and extend the thigh.

# Mock examinations

The following three mock examinations are set in the same format as the current exam. There are 20 images for each exam, and 75 minutes in which to answer them. The exam is undertaken on a digital viewing system, with a paper answer booklet. These mock exams mimic the same style. The answers are provided at the end of the mock exam.

# Mock examination 1

# Image 1

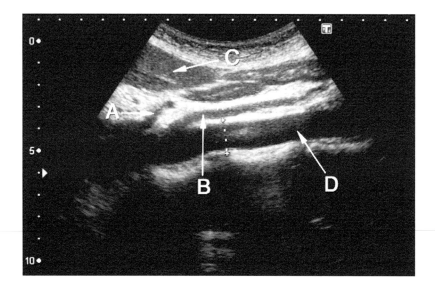

## QUESTIONS

A   Name the structure labelled A.
B   Name the structure labelled B.
C   Name the structure labelled C.
D   Name the structure labelled D.
E   What is the maximum normal measurement of D? (between the calipers labelled 'A')

# Image 2

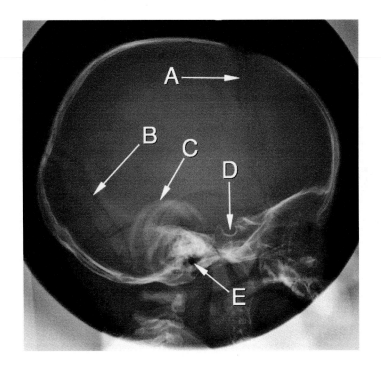

## QUESTIONS

A   Name the structure labelled A.
B   Name the structure labelled B.
C   Name the structure labelled C.
D   Name the structure labelled D.
E   Name the structure labelled E.

# Image 3

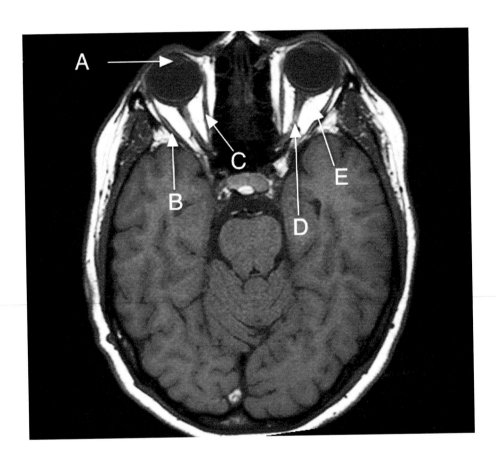

## QUESTIONS

A   Name the structure labelled A.
B   Name the structure labelled B.
C   Name the structure labelled C.
D   Name the structure labelled D.
E   Name the structure labelled E.

# Image 4

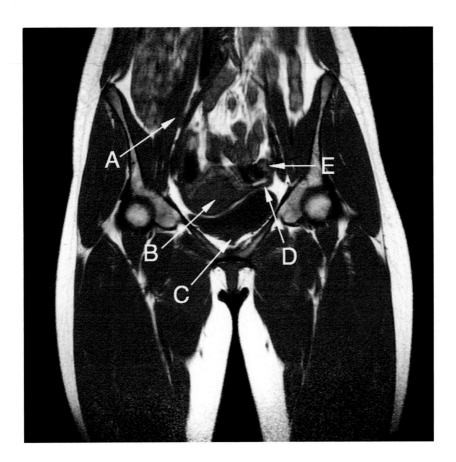

## QUESTIONS

A  Name the structure labelled A.
B  Name the structure labelled B.
C  Name the structure labelled C.
D  Name the structure labelled D.
E  Name the structure labelled E.

# Image 5

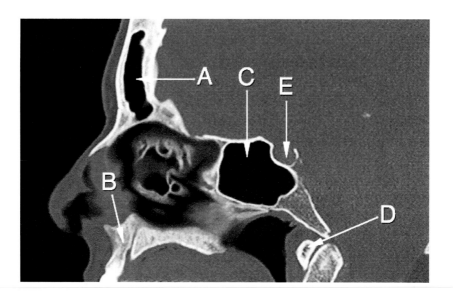

## QUESTIONS

A Name the structure labelled A.
B Name the structure labelled B.
C Name the structure labelled C.
D Name the structure labelled D.
E Name the structure labelled E.

# Image 6

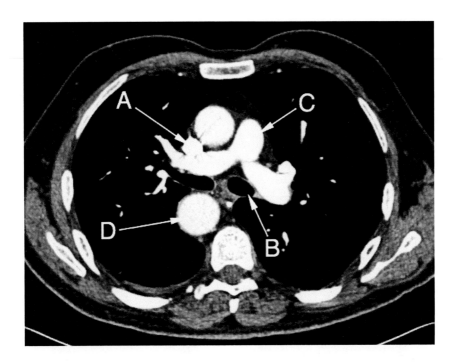

## QUESTIONS

A   Name the structure labelled A.
B   Name the structure labelled B.
C   Name the structure labelled C.
D   Name the structure labelled D.
E   What is the anatomical variant?

# Image 7

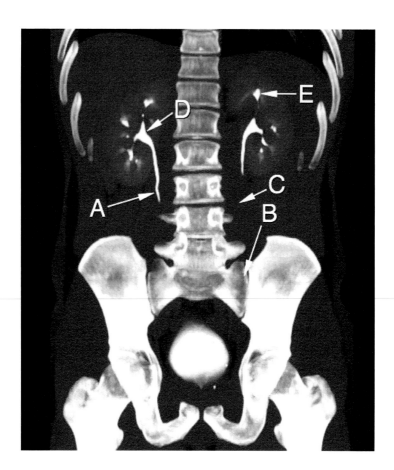

## QUESTIONS

A   Name the structure labelled A.
B   Name the structure labelled B.
C   Name the structure labelled C.
D   Name the structure labelled D.
E   Name the structure labelled E.

# Image 8

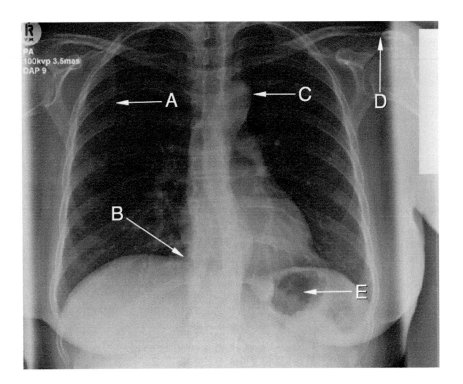

## QUESTIONS

A   Name the structure labelled A.
B   Name the structure labelled B.
C   Name the structure labelled C.
D   Name the structure labelled D.
E   Name the structure labelled E.

# Image 9

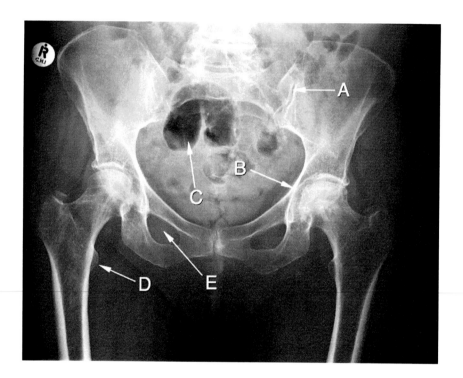

## QUESTIONS

A   Name the structure labelled A.
B   Name the structure labelled B.
C   Name the structure labelled C.
D   Name the structure labelled D.
E   Name the structure labelled E.

# Image 10

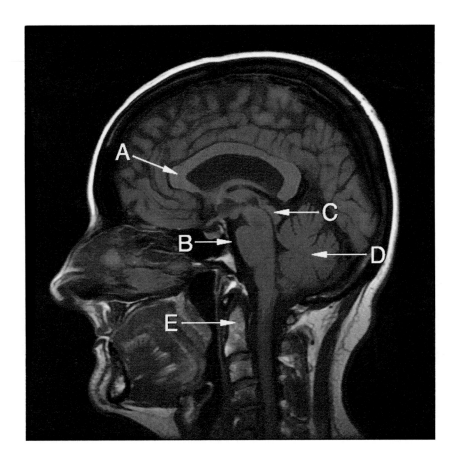

## QUESTIONS

A   Name the structure labelled A.
B   Name the structure labelled B.
C   Name the structure labelled C.
D   Name the structure labelled D.
E   Name the structure labelled E.

# Image 11

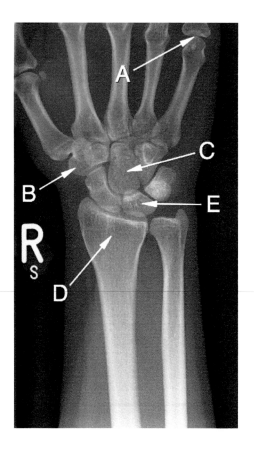

## QUESTIONS

A   Name the structure labelled A.
B   Name the structure labelled B.
C   Name the structure labelled C.
D   Name the structure labelled D.
E   Name the structure labelled E.

# Image 12

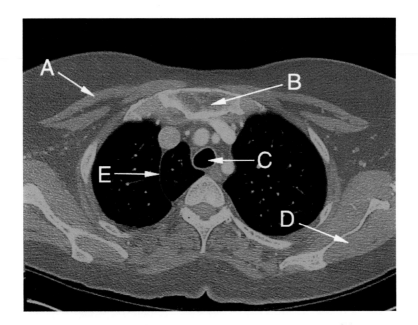

## QUESTIONS

A   Name the structure labelled A.
B   Name the structure labelled B.
C   Name the structure labelled C.
D   Name the structure labelled D.
E   Name the anatomical variant labelled E.

# Image 13

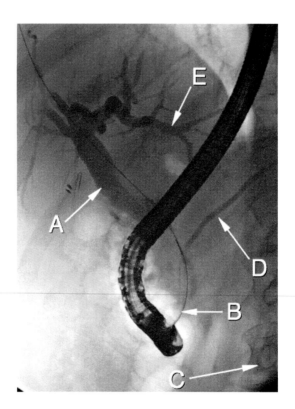

## QUESTIONS

A   Name the structure labelled A.
B   Name the structure labelled B.
C   Name the structure labelled C.
D   Name the structure labelled D.
E   Name the structure labelled E.

# Image 14

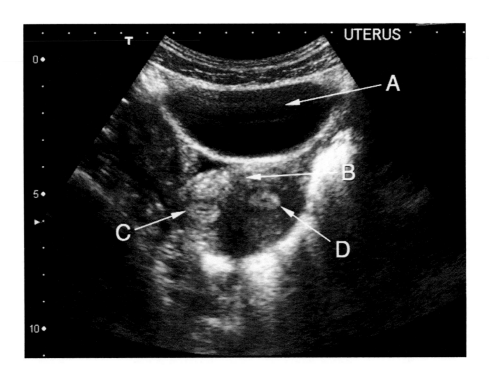

## QUESTIONS

A   Name the structure labelled A.
B   Name the structure labelled B.
C   Name the structure labelled C.
D   Name the structure labelled D.
E   Name an anatomical variant that this may represent.

# Image 15

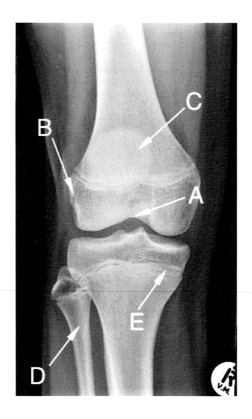

## QUESTIONS

A    Name the structure labelled A.
B    Name the structure labelled B.
C    Name the structure labelled C.
D    Name the structure labelled D.
E    Name the structure labelled E.

# Image 16

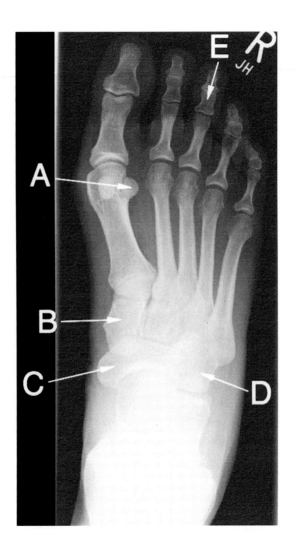

## QUESTIONS

A   Name the structure labelled A.
B   Name the structure labelled B.
C   Name the structure labelled C.
D   Name the structure labelled D.
E   Name the structure labelled E.

# Image 17

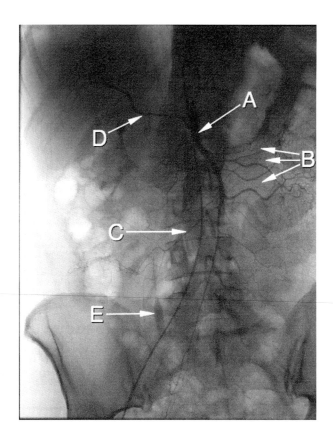

## QUESTIONS

A   Name the structure labelled A.
B   Name the structure labelled B.
C   Name the structure labelled C.
D   Name the structure labelled D.
E   Name the structure labelled E.

# Image 18

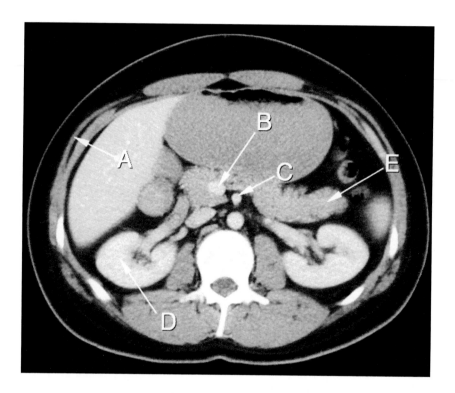

## QUESTIONS

A Name the structure labelled A.
B Name the structure labelled B.
C Name the structure labelled C.
D Name the structure labelled D.
E Name the structure labelled E.

# Image 19

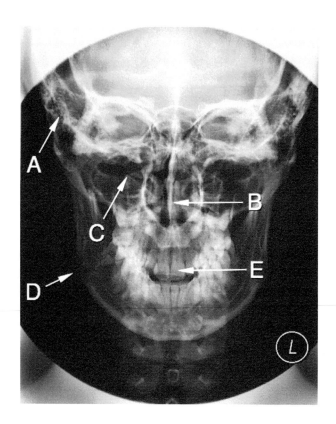

## QUESTIONS

A   Name the structure labelled A.
B   Name the structure labelled B.
C   Name the structure labelled C.
D   Name the structure labelled D.
E   Name the structure labelled E.

# Image 20

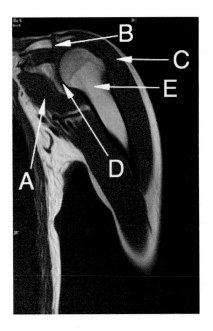

## QUESTIONS

A   Name the structure labelled A.
B   Name the structure labelled B.
C   Name the structure labelled C.
D   Name the structure labelled D.
E   Name the structure labelled E.

# MOCK EXAMINATION 1: ANSWERS

**M1.1**

A   Coeliac axis
B   Superior mesenteric artery
C   Liver
D   Abdominal aorta
E   3 cm


**M1.2**

A   Coronal suture
B   Lambdoid suture
C   Pinna of ear
D   Sella turcica/pituitary fossa
E   External acoustic meatus


**M1.3**

A   Right lens of globe
B   Right lateral rectus
C   Right medial rectus
D   Left optic nerve
E   Intraconal fat


**M1.4**

A   Right psoas muscle
B   Uterus
C   Bladder neck
D   Left broad ligament
E   Left ovary


**M1.5**

A   Frontal sinus
B   Maxilla
C   Sphenoid sinus
D   Anterior arch of C1
E   Sella turcica/pituitary fossa

## M1.6

A   Superior vena cava
B   Left main bronchus
C   Main pulmonary artery
D   Descending thoracic aorta
E   A right-sided aortic arch

## M1.7

A   Right ureter
B   Left sacroiliac joint
C   Left psoas muscle
D   Right renal pelvis
E   Left upper pole calyx

## M1.8

A   Medial border of right scapula
B   Right cardiophrenic angle
C   Aortic knuckle
D   Left acromioclavicular joint
E   Gastric bubble

## M1.9

A   Left sacroiliac joint
B   Left acetabulum
C   Sigmoid colon
D   Right lesser trochanter
E   Right obturator foramen

## M1.10

A   Genu of corpus callosum
B   Prepontine cistern
C   Quadrigeminal plate
D   Cerebellum
E   Odontoid peg

## M1.11

A   Metacarpophalangeal joint of little finger
B   Trapezium
C   Capitate
D   Head of radius
E   Lunate

## M1.12
A   Right pectoralis major
B   Manubrium
C   Trachea
D   Left infraspinatus
E   Azygos fissure

## M1.13
A   Common bile duct
B   Ampulla of Vater
C   Lumbar vertebrae pedicle
D   Main pancreatic duct
E   Left intrahepatic duct

## M1.14
A   Bladder
B   Uterus
C   Uterine cavity
D   Uterine cavity
E   Bicornuate uterus/septate uterus/didelphys

## M1.15
A   Intercondylar fossa
B   Lateral femoral condyle
C   Patella
D   Neck of fibula
E   Epiphyseal line

## M1.16
A   Sesamoid bone in flexor hallucis brevis muscle
B   Right medial cuneiform
C   Right navicular
D   Right cuboid
E   Right middle phalanx of third toe

## M1.17
A   Superior mesenteric artery
B   Jejunal branches
C   Ileocolic branch
D   Replaced/additional right hepatic artery
E   Right ureter

**M1.18**
A   Right external oblique
B   Superior mesenteric vein
C   Superior mesenteric artery
D   Right kidney
E   Tail of pancreas


**M1.19**
A   Right mastoid air cells
B   Nasal septum
C   Right superior orbital fissure
D   Right angle of mandible
E   Upper medial incisor


**M1.20**
A   Subscapularis
B   Acromioclavicular joint
C   Deltoid
D   Glenohumeral joint
E   Surgical neck of the humerus

# Mock examination 2

## Image 1

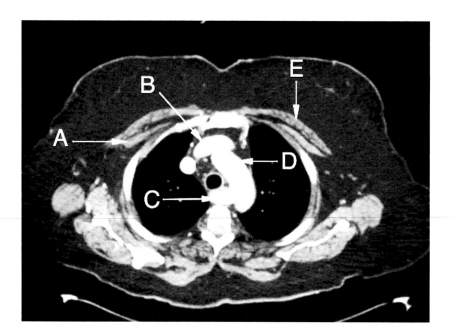

### QUESTIONS

A    Name the structure labelled A.
B    Name the structure labelled B.
C    Name the anatomical variant labelled C.
D    Name the structure labelled D.
E    Name the structure labelled E.

# Image 2

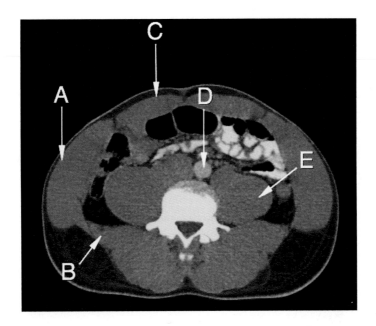

## QUESTIONS

A    Name the structure labelled A.
B    Name the structure labelled B.
C    Name the structure labelled C.
D    Name the structure labelled D.
E    Name the structure labelled E.

# Image 3

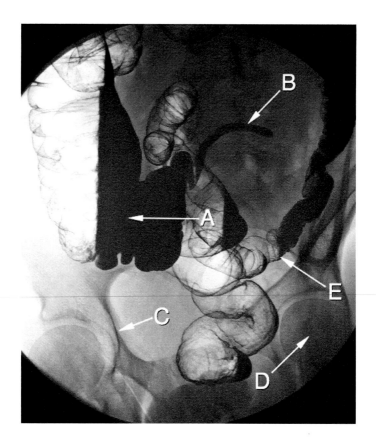

## QUESTIONS

A    Name the structure labelled A.
B    Name the structure labelled B.
C    Name the structure labelled C.
D    Name the structure labelled D.
E    Name the structure labelled E.

# Image 4

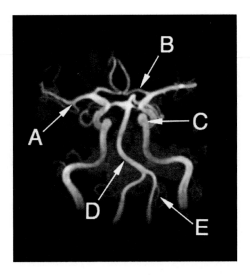

## QUESTIONS

A   Name the structure labelled A.
B   Name the anatomical variant labelled B.
C   Name the structure labelled C.
D   Name the structure labelled D.
E   Name the structure labelled E.

# Image 5

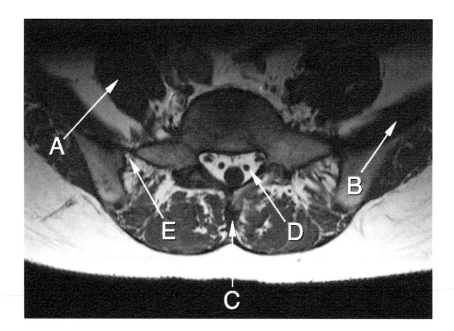

## QUESTIONS

A  Name the structure labelled A.
B  Name the structure labelled B.
C  Name the structure labelled C.
D  Name the structure labelled D.
E  Name the structure labelled E.

# Image 6

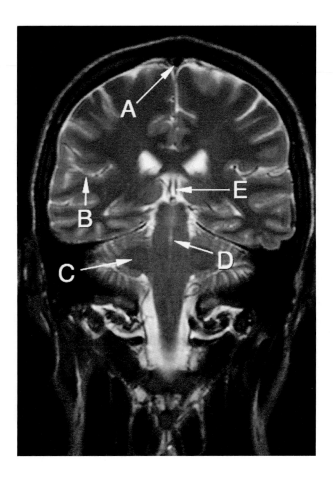

## QUESTIONS

A   Name the structure labelled A.
B   Name the structure labelled B.
C   Name the structure labelled C.
D   Name the structure labelled D.
E   Name the structure labelled E.

# Image 7

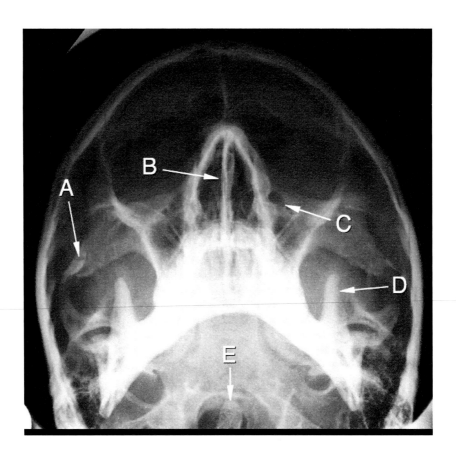

## QUESTIONS

A  Name the structure labelled A.
B  Name the structure labelled B.
C  Name the structure labelled C.
D  Name the structure labelled D.
E  Name the structure labelled E.

# Image 8

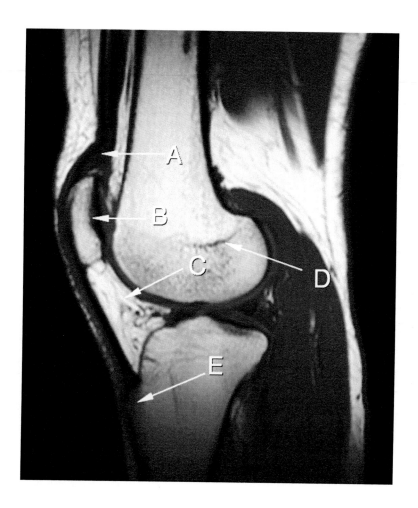

## QUESTIONS

A   Name the structure labelled A.
B   Name the structure labelled B.
C   Name the structure labelled C.
D   Name the structure labelled D.
E   Name the structure labelled E.

# Image 9

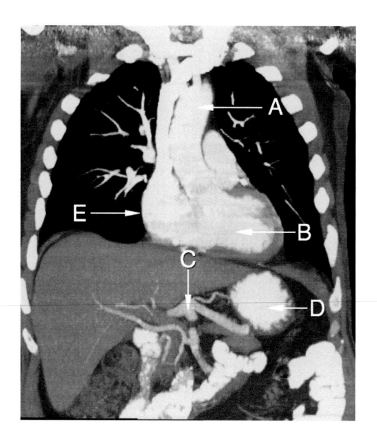

## QUESTIONS

A   Name the structure labelled A.
B   Name the structure labelled B.
C   Name the structure labelled C.
D   Name the structure labelled D.
E   Name the structure labelled E.

# Image 10

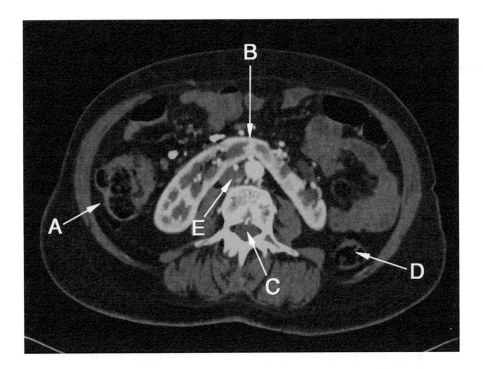

## QUESTIONS

A   Name the structure labelled A.
B   Name the anatomical variant labelled B.
C   Name the structure labelled C.
D   Name the structure labelled D.
E   Name the structure labelled E.

# Image 11

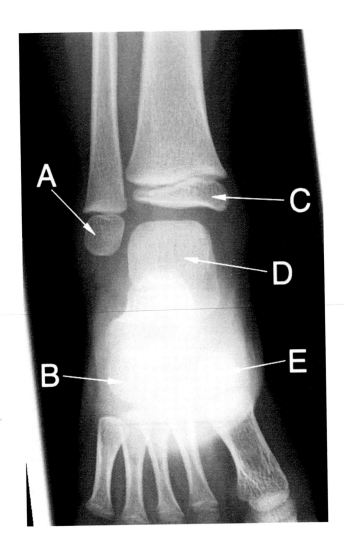

## QUESTIONS

A   Name the structure labelled A.
B   Name the structure labelled B.
C   Name the structure labelled C.
D   Name the structure labelled D.
E   Name the structure labelled E.

# Image 12

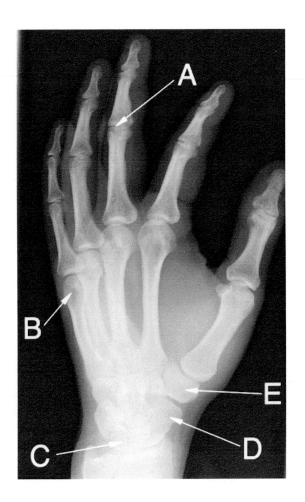

## QUESTIONS

A    Name the structure labelled A.
B    Name the structure labelled B.
C    Name the structure labelled C.
D    Name the structure labelled D.
E    Name the structure labelled E.

# Image 13

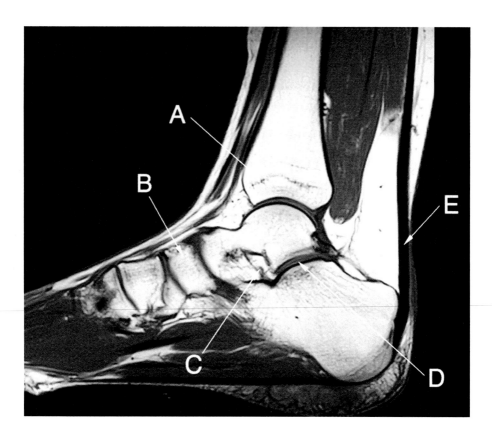

## QUESTIONS

A   Name the structure labelled A.
B   Name the structure labelled B.
C   Name the structure labelled C.
D   Name the structure labelled D.
E   Name the structure labelled E.

# Image 14

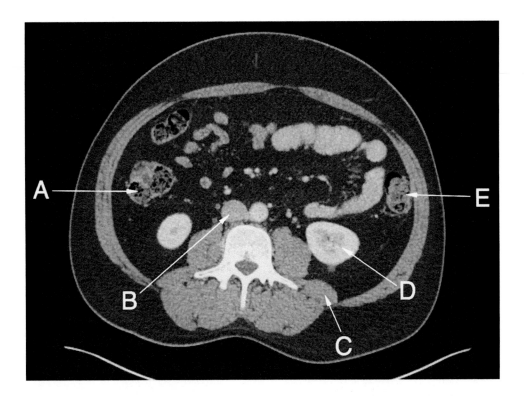

## QUESTIONS

A   Name the structure labelled A.
B   Name the structure labelled B.
C   Name the structure labelled C.
D   Name the structure labelled D.
E   Name the structure labelled E.

# Image 15

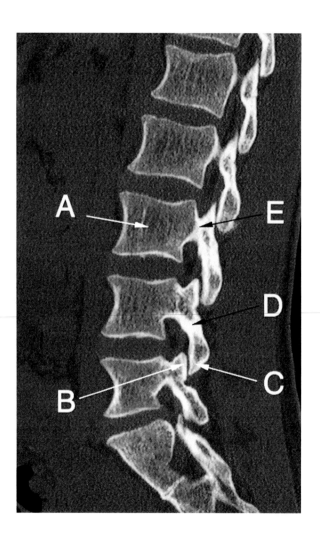

## QUESTIONS

A   Name the structure labelled A.
B   Name the structure labelled B.
C   Name the structure labelled C.
D   Name the structure labelled D.
E   Name the structure labelled E.

# Image 16

This is a volume-rendered reconstruction of the heart and great vessels.

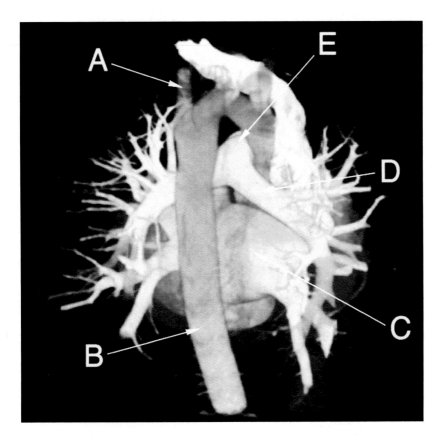

## QUESTIONS

A   Name the structure labelled A.
B   Name the structure labelled B.
C   Name the structure labelled C.
D   Name the structure labelled D.
E   Name the structure labelled E.

# Image 17

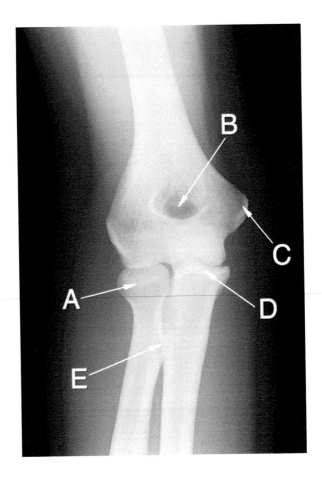

## QUESTIONS

A   Name the structure labelled A.
B   Name the structure labelled B.
C   Name the structure labelled C.
D   Name the structure labelled D.
E   Which upper limb muscle has part of its tendinous attachment at this point?

# Image 18

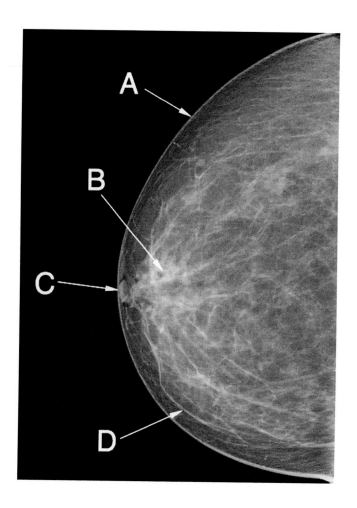

## QUESTIONS

A  Name the structure labelled A.
B  Name the structure labelled B.
C  Name the structure labelled C.
D  Name the structure labelled D.
E  What is the name of this projection?

# Image 19

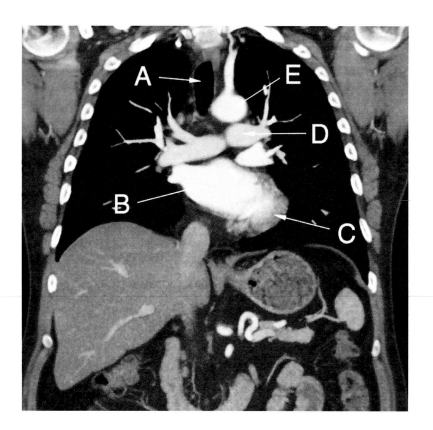

## QUESTIONS

A   Name the structure labelled A.
B   Name the structure labelled B.
C   Name the structure labelled C.
D   Name the structure labelled D.
E   Name the structure labelled E.

# Image 20

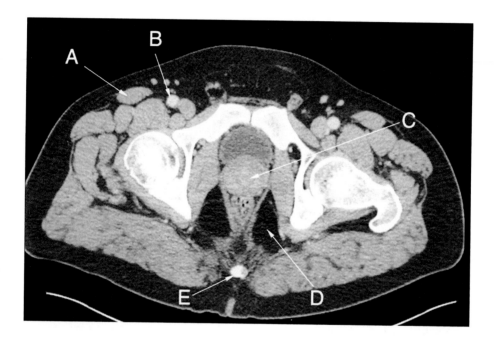

## QUESTIONS

A  Name the structure labelled A.
B  Name the structure labelled B.
C  Name the structure labelled C.
D  Name the structure labelled D.
E  Name the structure labelled E.

# MOCK EXAMINATION 2: ANSWERS

**M2.1**
A   Right pectoralis minor
B   Left brachiocephalic vein
C   Aberrant right subclavian artery
D   Aortic arch
E   Left pectoralis major

**M2.2**
A   Right external oblique
B   Right quadratus lumborum
C   Right rectus abdominis
D   Aorta
E   Left psoas

**M2.3**
A   Caecum
B   Appendix
C   Right acetabulum
D   Left femoral head
E   Sigmoid colon

**M2.4**
A   Genu of middle cerebral artery
B   A2 – anterior cerebral artery
C   Cavernous portion of internal carotid artery
D   Basilar artery
E   Left posterior inferior cerebellar artery

**M2.5**
A   Right psoas
B   Left iliacus
C   Spinous process
D   Spinal nerve root
E   Right sacroiliac joint

**M2.6**
A    Superior sagittal sinus
B    Right Sylvian fissure
C    Middle cerebellar peduncle
D    Aqueduct of Sylvius
E    Internal cerebral veins


**M2.7**
A    Right zygomatic arch
B    Nasal septum
C    Left infraorbital fissure
D    Left coronoid process
E    Odontoid peg


**M2.8**
A    Quadriceps tendon
B    Patella
C    Infrapatellar fat pad
D    Epiphyseal scar
E    Tibial tuberosity


**M2.9**
A    Ascending aorta
B    Left ventricle
C    Coeliac axis
D    Stomach
E    Right atrium


**M2.10**
A    Ascending colon
B    Horseshoe kidney
C    Spinal cord
D    Descending colon
E    Inferior vena cava


**M2.11**
A    Ossification centre for distal fibula
B    Cuboid
C    Ossification centre for distal tibia
D    Talus
E    Medial cuneiform

## M2.12
A  Middle finger proximal interphalangeal joint
B  Head of little finger metacarpal
C  Lunate
D  Scaphoid
E  Trapezium

## M2.13
A  Distal tibia
B  Navicular
C  Sinus tarsi
D  Subtalar joint (posterior)
E  Achilles tendon/tendo calcaneus

## M2.14
A  Ascending colon
B  Inferior vena cava
C  Left quadratus lumborum
D  Left kidney
E  Descending colon

## M2.15
A  Body of third lumbar vertebra
B  Superior facet of fifth lumbar vertebra
C  Inferior facet of fourth lumbar vertebra
D  Pars interarticularis of fourth lumbar vertebra
E  Pedicle of third lumbar vertebra

## M2.16
A  Left subclavian artery
B  Descending aorta
C  Left atrium
D  Right pulmonary artery
E  Pulmonary trunk/main pulmonary artery

## M2.17
A  Radial head
B  Olecranon fossa
C  Medial epicondyle of humerus
D  Coronoid process of ulna
E  Biceps brachii (at radial tuberosity)

**M2.18**
A  Skin
B  Glandular tissue
C  Nipple
D  Suspensory ligament of Cooper
E  Cranio-caudal (CC)


**M2.19**
A  Trachea
B  Left atrium
C  Left ventricle
D  Left pulmonary artery
E  Aortic arch


**M2.20**
A  Right sartorius
B  Right common femoral artery
C  Prostate
D  Left ischio-rectal/anal fossa
E  Coccyx

# Mock examination 3

## Image 1

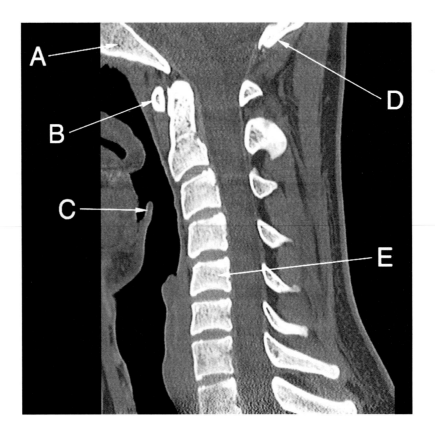

**QUESTIONS**

A Name the structure labelled A.
B Name the structure labelled B.
C Name the structure labelled C.
D Name the structure labelled D.
E Name the structure labelled E.

# Image 2

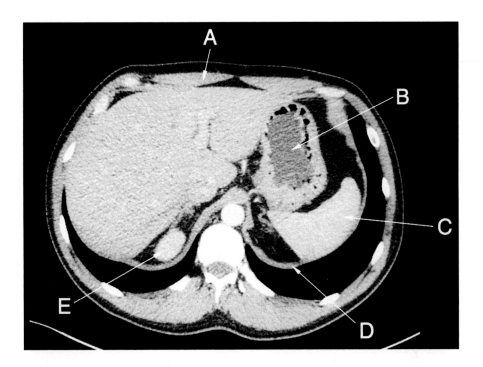

## QUESTIONS

A   Name the structure labelled A.
B   Name the structure labelled B.
C   Name the structure labelled C.
D   Name the structure labelled D.
E   Name the structure labelled E.

# Image 3

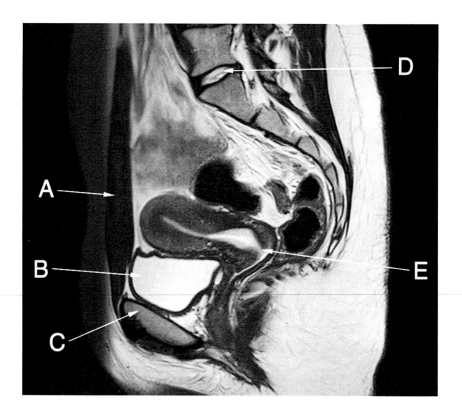

## QUESTIONS

A  Name the structure labelled A.
B  Name the structure labelled B.
C  Name the structure labelled C.
D  Name the structure labelled D.
E  Name the structure labelled E.

# Image 4

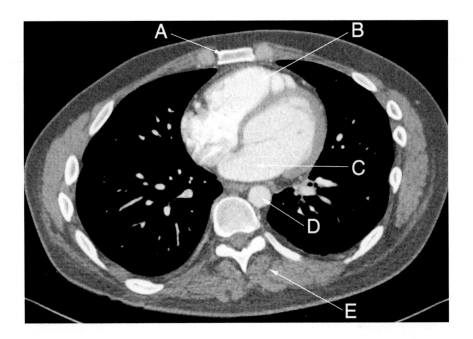

## QUESTIONS

A   Name the structure labelled A.
B   Name the structure labelled B.
C   Name the structure labelled C.
D   Name the structure labelled D.
E   Name the structure labelled E.

# Image 5

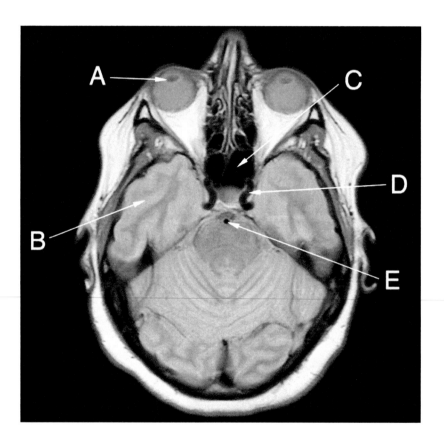

**QUESTIONS**

A   Name the structure labelled A.
B   Name the structure labelled B.
C   Name the structure labelled C.
D   Name the structure labelled D.
E   Name the structure labelled E.

# Image 6

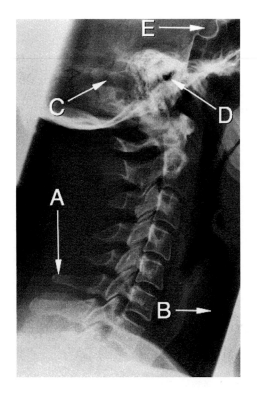

## QUESTIONS

A   Name the structure labelled A.
B   Name the structure labelled B.
C   Name the structure labelled C.
D   Name the structure labelled D.
E   Name the structure labelled E.

# Image 7

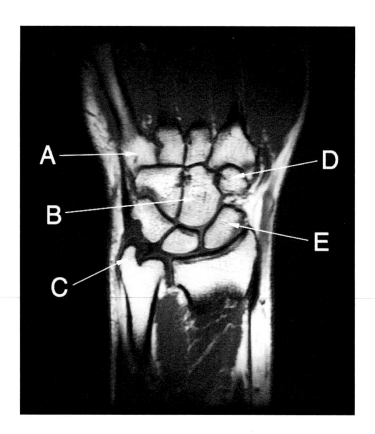

## QUESTIONS

A   Name the structure labelled A.
B   Name the structure labelled B.
C   Name the structure labelled C.
D   Name the structure labelled D.
E   Name the structure labelled E.

# Image 8

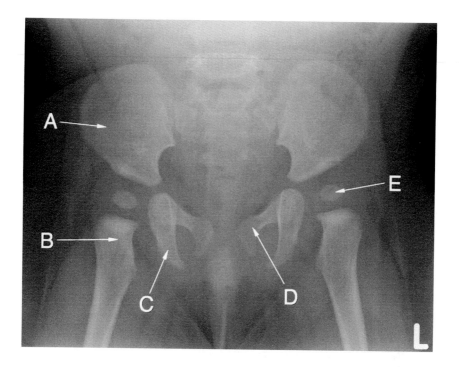

## QUESTIONS

A   Name the structure labelled A.
B   Name the structure labelled B.
C   Name the structure labelled C.
D   Name the structure labelled D.
E   Name the structure labelled E.

# Image 9

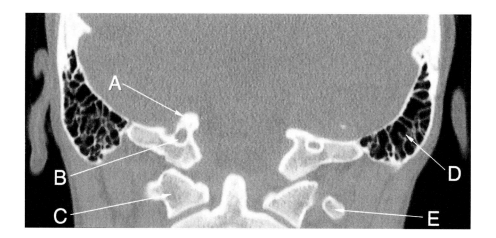

## QUESTIONS

A   Name the structure labelled A.
B   Name the structure labelled B.
C   Name the structure labelled C.
D   Name the structure labelled D.
E   Name the structure labelled E.

# Image 10

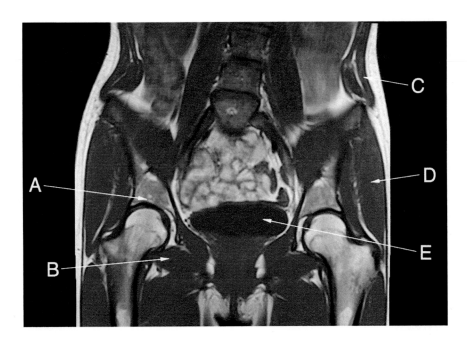

## QUESTIONS

A   Name the structure labelled A.
B   Name the structure labelled B.
C   Name the structure labelled C.
D   Name the structure labelled D.
E   Name the structure labelled E.

# Image 11

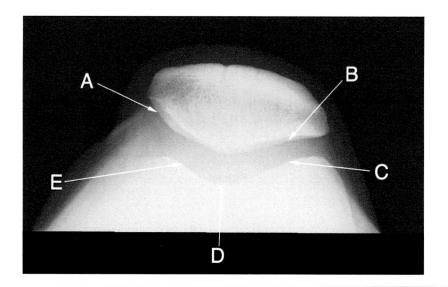

## QUESTIONS

A   Name the structure labelled A.
B   Name the structure labelled B.
C   Name the structure labelled C.
D   Name the structure labelled D.
E   Name the structure labelled E.

# Image 12

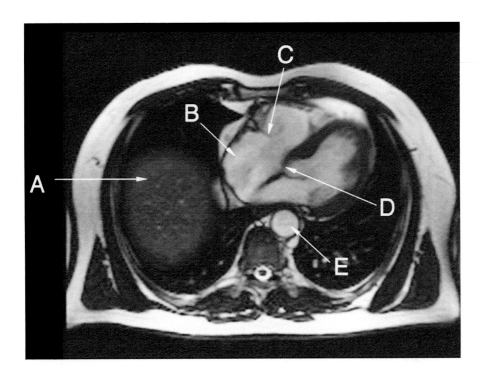

## QUESTIONS

A   Name the structure labelled A.
B   Name the structure labelled B.
C   Name the structure labelled C.
D   Name the structure labelled D.
E   Name the structure labelled E.

# Image 13

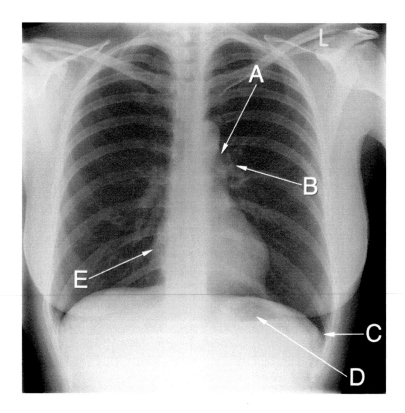

## QUESTIONS

A  What is the name of this potential space?
B  Name the structure labelled B.
C  Name the structure labelled C.
D  Within which structure does this lie?
E  To which part of the heart does this margin relate?

# Image 14

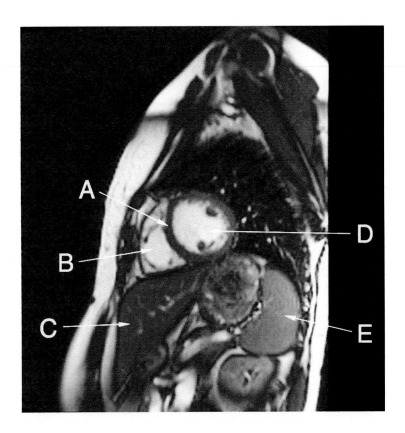

## QUESTIONS

A  Name the structure labelled A.
B  Name the structure labelled B.
C  Name the structure labelled C.
D  Name the structure labelled D.
E  Name the structure labelled E.

# Image 15

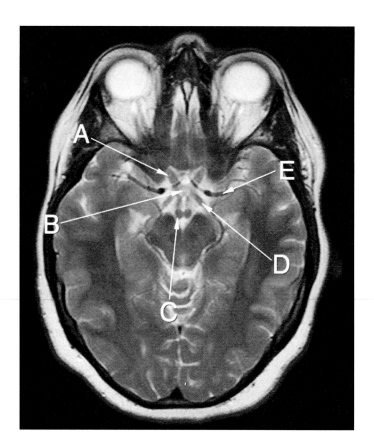

## QUESTIONS

A   Name the structure labelled A.
B   Name the structure labelled B.
C   Name the structure labelled C.
D   Name the structure labelled D.
E   Name the structure labelled E.

# Image 16

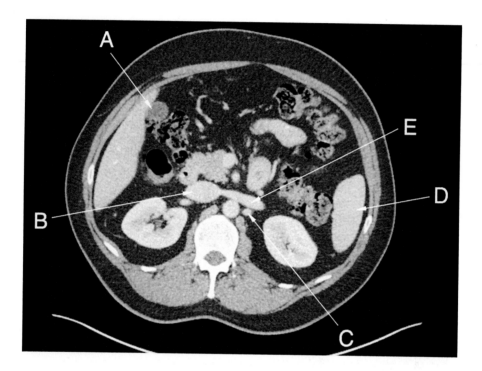

## QUESTIONS

A   Name the structure labelled A.
B   Name the structure labelled B.
C   Name the structure labelled C.
D   Name the structure labelled D.
E   Name the structure labelled E.

# Image 17

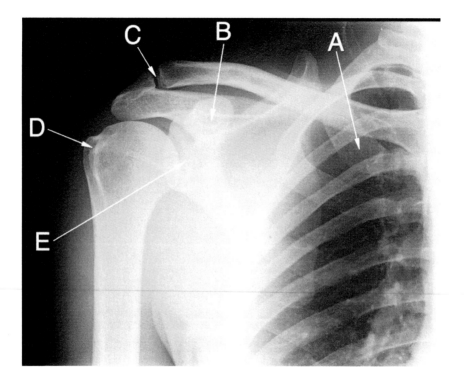

## QUESTIONS

A   Name the structure labelled A.
B   Name the structure labelled B.
C   Name the structure labelled C.
D   Which three rotator cuff muscles attach at point D?
E   Name the structure labelled E.

# Image 18

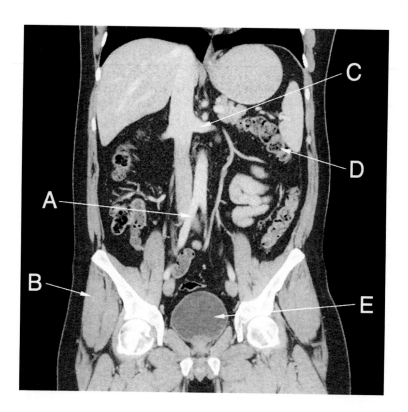

## QUESTIONS

A   Name the structure labelled A.
B   Name the structure labelled B.
C   Name the structure labelled C.
D   Name the structure labelled D.
E   Name the structure labelled E.

# Image 19

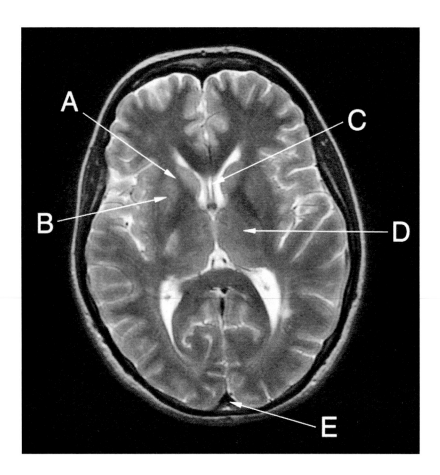

## QUESTIONS

A   Name the structure labelled A.
B   Name the structure labelled B.
C   Name the structure labelled C.
D   Name the structure labelled D.
E   Name the structure labelled E.

# Image 20

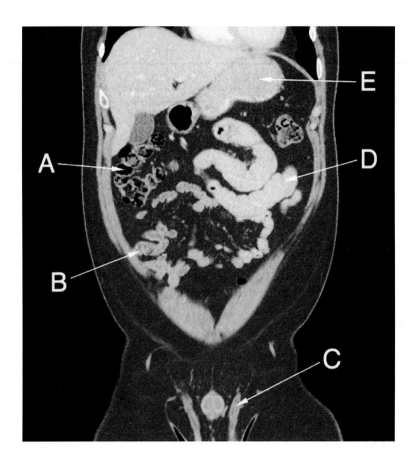

**QUESTIONS**

A   Name the structure labelled A.
B   Name the structure labelled B.
C   Name the structure labelled C.
D   Name the structure labelled D.
E   Name the structure labelled E.

# MOCK EXAMINATION 3: ANSWERS

**M3.1**
A   Clivus
B   Anterior arch of atlas (C1)
C   Epiglottis
D   Occiput
E   Body of fifth cervical vertebra (C5)

**M3.2**
A   Right rectus abdominis
B   Stomach
C   Spleen
D   Left hemidiaphragm
E   Right kidney

**M3.3**
A   Rectus abdominis
B   Bladder
C   Pubic symphysis/pubis
D   Intervertebral disc at L5/S1 level
E   Cervix of uterus

**M3.4**
A   Sternum
B   Right ventricle/ventricular cavity
C   Left atrium/atrial cavity
D   Descending thoracic aorta
E   Erector spinae

**M3.5**
A   Lens of right globe
B   Right temporal lobe
C   Sphenoid sinus
D   Cavernous segment of left internal carotid artery
E   Basilar artery

**M3.6**
A   Spinous process of C6
B   Trachea
C   Pinna of ear
D   External acoustic meatus
E   Sella turcica/pituitary fossa

**M3.7**
A   Base of little finger metacarpal
B   Capitate
C   Ulnar styloid
D   Trapezoid
E   Scaphoid

**M3.8**
A   Right ilium
B   Right neck of femur
C   Right ischium
D   Left pubis
E   Ossification centre for left capital femoral epiphysis

**M3.9**
A   Right jugular tubercle
B   Right hypoglossal canal
C   Right lateral mass of atlas (C1)
D   Left mastoid air cells
E   Left transverse process of atlas (C1)

**M3.10**
A   Right acetabulum
B   Right obturator externus
C   Left external oblique
D   Left gluteus medius
E   Bladder

**M3.11**
A   Medial facet of patella
B   Lateral facet of patella
C   Lateral condyle of femur
D   Trochlear groove
E   Medial condyle of femur

## M3.12
A    Right lobe of liver
B    Right atrium
C    Tricuspid valve
D    Membranous interventricular septum
E    Descending thoracic aorta

## M3.13
A    Aorto-pulmonary window
B    Left pulmonary artery
C    Left costophrenic angle
D    Stomach
E    Right atrium

## M3.14
A    Muscular interventricular septum
B    Right ventricle/ventricular cavity
C    Left lobe of liver
D    Spleen
E    Left ventricle/ventricular cavity

## M3.15
A    Right optic nerve
B    Optic chiasm or pituitary gland
C    Right mammillary body
D    Left optic tract
E    Left middle cerebral artery

## M3.16
A    Gallbladder
B    Inferior vena cava
C    Left renal artery
D    Spleen
E    Left renal vein

## M3.17
A    Right first rib
B    Coracoid process
C    Acromioclavicular joint
D    Supraspinatus, infraspinatus and teres minor
E    Glenoid fossa

**M3.18**

A    Right common iliac artery
B    Right gluteus medius
C    Left renal vein
D    Splenic flexure/descending colon
E    Bladder

**M3.19**

A    Right internal capsule
B    Right lentiform nucleus (globus pallidus/putamen)
C    Septum pellucidum
D    Left thalamus
E    Superior sagittal sinus

**M3.20**

A    Hepatic flexure/ascending colon
B    Ileum
C    Left spermatic cord
D    Jejunum
E    Stomach

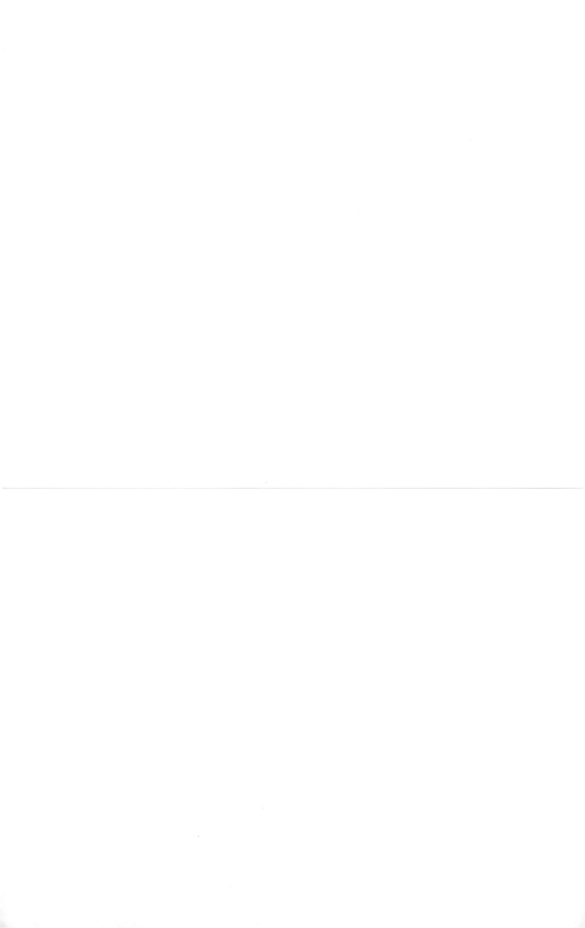

# Index